# Scar Revision

## Procedures in Cosmetic Dermatology

**Series Editor: Jeffrey S. Dover MD FRCPC**
**Associate Editor: Murad Alam MD**

**Botulinum Toxin**
*Alastair Carruthers MABM BCh FRCPC FRCP(Lon) and*
*Jean Carruthers MD FRCS(C) FRC(OPHTH)*
*ISBN 1 4160 2470 0*

**Soft Tissue Augmentation**
*Jean Carruthers MD FRCS(C) FRC(OPHTH) and*
*Alastair Carruthers MABM BCh FRCPC FRCP(Lon)*
*ISBN 1 4160 2469 7*

**Cosmeceuticals**
*Zoe Diana Draelos MD*
*ISBN 1 4160 0244 8*

**Laser and Lights: Volume 1**
**Vascular • Pigmentation • Scars • Medical Applications**
*David J. Goldberg MD JD*
*ISBN 1 4160 2386 0*

**Laser and Lights: Volume 2**
**Rejuvenation • Resurfacing • Hair Removal • Treatment of Ethnic Skin**
*David J. Goldberg MD JD*
*ISBN 1 4160 2387 9*

**Photodynamic Therapy**
*Mitchel P. Goldman MD*
*ISBN 1 4160 2360 7*

**Liposuction**
*C. William Hanke MD MPH FACP and Gerhard Sattler MD*
*ISBN 1 4160 22082*

**Scar Revision**
*Kenneth A. Arndt MD*
*ISBN 1 4160 31316*

**Chemical Peels**
*Mark Rubin MD*
*ISBN 1 4160 30719*

**Hair Transplantation**
*Dowling B. Stough MD and Robert S. Haber MD*
*ISBN 1 4160 31049*

**Leg Veins**
*Murad Alam MD and Tri H. Nguyen MD*
*ISBN 1 4160 31596*

**Blepharoplasty**
*Ronald L. Moy MD and Edgar F. Fincher MD PhD*
*ISBN 1 4160 29966*

**Advance Face Lifting**
*Ronald L. Moy MD and Edgar F. Fincher MD PhD*
*ISBN 1 4160 29974*

PROCEDURES IN COSMETIC DERMATOLOGY

Series Editor: Jeffrey S. Dover MD FRCPC

Associate Editor: Murad Alam MD

# Scar Revision

Edited by

**Kenneth A. Arndt** MD

Clinical Professor of Dermatology, Yale University School of Medicine; Adjunct Professor of Medicine (Dermatology), Dartmouth Medical School; Clinical Professor of Medicine, Harvard Medical School; Director, SkinCare Physicians of Chestnut Hill, Chestnut Hill, MA, USA

Series Editor

**Jeffrey S. Dover** MD FRCPC

Associate Professor of Clinical Dermatology, Yale University School of Medicine; Adjunct Professor of Medicine (Dermatology), Dartmouth Medical School; Director, SkinCare Physicians of Chestnut Hill, Chestnut Hill, MA, USA

Associate Editor

**Murad Alam** MD

Chief, Section of Cutaneous and Aesthetic Surgery, Departments of Dermatology and Otolaryngology-Head and Neck Surgery, Northwestern University, Chicago, IL USA

ELSEVIER
SAUNDERS

ELSEVIER
SAUNDERS

An imprint of Elsevier Inc.

First published 2006



ISBN: 1 4160 31316

**British Library Cataloguing in Publication Data**
A catalogue record for this book is available from the British Library

**Library of Congress Cataloging in Publication Data**
A catalog record for this book is available from the Library of Congress

**Notice**

Medical knowledge is constantly changing. Standard safety precautions must be followed, but as new research and clinical experience broaden our knowledge, changes in treatment and drug therapy may become necessary or appropriate. Readers are advised to check the most current product information provided by the manufacturer of each drug to be administered to verify the recommended dose, the method and duration of administration, and contraindications. It is the responsibility of the practitioner, relying on experience and knowledge of the patient, to determine dosages and the best treatment for each individual patient. Neither the Publisher nor the editor assumes any liability for any injury and/or damage to persons or property arising from this publication.

**The Publisher**

Printed in China
Last digit is the print number: 9 8 7 6 5 4 3 2 1



Commissioning Editor: **Karen Bowler**
Project Development Managers: **Martin Mellor Publishing Services Ltd, Seán Duggan, Louise Cook**
Project Managers: **Naughton Project Management, Cheryl Brant**
Illustration Managers: **Mick Ruddy, Gillian Murray**
Design Manager: **Andy Chapman**
Illustrators: **Richard Prime, Tim Loughhead**

# Contents


**Series Foreword** vii

**Preface** ix

**List of Contributors** xi

1 **What are Scars?** 1
*Bahar Dasgeb, Tania J. Phillips*

2 **The Medical Treatment of Scarring** 17
*Brian Berman, Deborah Zell*

3 **Surgical Approaches to Patients with Scarring** 45
*Joanna Mimi Choi, Thomas E. Rohrer, Michael S. Kaminer, R. Sonia Batra*

4 **Treatment of Scars with Lasers and Other Energy Sources** 67
*Keyvan Nouri, Maria Patricia Rivas, Christopher J. Ballard*

5 **Effect of Radiation on Wound Healing and the Treatment of Scarring** 89
*Roy H. Decker, Lynn D. Wilson*

6 **Laser-induced Repigmentation of Scars** 105
*Roy G. Geronemus, Galen H. Fisher*

7 **Special Considerations in the Approach to Treatment and Management of Scars in African-Americans and Other Populations More at Risk** 115
*A. Paul Kelly*

8 **Camouflage Therapy for Scars** 123
*Neil Shear*

**Index** 135

# Series Foreword
## Procedures in Cosmetic Dermatology

While dermatologists have been procedurally inclined since the beginning of the specialty, particularly rapid change has occurred in the past quarter century. The advent of frozen section technique and the golden age of Mohs skin cancer surgery has led to the formal incorporation of surgery within the dermatology curriculum. More recently technological breakthroughs in minimally invasive procedural dermatology have offered an aging population new options for improving the appearance of damaged skin.

Procedures for rejuvenating the skin and adjacent regions are actively sought by our patients. Significantly, dermatologists have pioneered devices, technologies and medications, which have continued to evolve at a startling pace. Numerous major advances, including virtually all cutaneous lasers and light-source based procedures, botulinum exotoxin, soft-tissue augmentation, dilute anesthesia liposuction, leg vein treatments, chemical peels, and hair transplants, have been invented, or developed and enhanced by dermatologists. Dermatologists understand procedures, and we have special insight into the structure, function, and working of skin. Cosmetic dermatologists have made rejuvenation accessible to risk-averse patients by emphasizing safety and reducing operative trauma. No specialty is better positioned than dermatology to lead the field of cutaneous surgery while meeting patient needs.

As dermatology grows as a specialty, an ever-increasing proportion of dermatologists will become proficient in the delivery of different procedures. Not all dermatologists will perform all procedures, and some will perform very few, but even the less procedurally directed amongst us must be well-versed in the details to be able to guide and educate our patients. Whether you are a skilled dermatologic surgeon interested in further expanding your surgical repertoire, a complete surgical novice wishing to learn a few simple procedures, or somewhere in between, this book and this series is for you.

The volume you are holding is one of a series entitled "Procedures in Cosmetic Dermatology." The purpose of each book is to serve as a practical primer on a major topic area in procedural dermatology.

If you want make sure you find the right book for your needs, you may wish to know what this book is and what it is not. It is not a comprehensive text grounded in theoretical underpinnings. It is not exhaustively referenced. It is not designed to be a completely unbiased review of the world's literature on the subject. At the same time, it is not an overview of cosmetic procedures that describes these in generalities without providing enough specific information to actually permit someone to perform the procedures. And importantly, it is not so heavy that it can serve as a doorstop or a shelf filler.

What this book and this series offer is a step-by-step, practical guide to performing cutaneous surgical procedures. Each volume in the series has been edited by a known authority in that subfield. Each editor has recruited other equally practical-minded, technically skilled, hands-on clinicians to write the constituent chapters. Most chapters have two authors to ensure that different approaches and a broad range of opinions are incorporated. On the other hand, the two authors and the editors also collectively provide a consistency of tone. A uniform template has been used within each chapter so that the reader will be easily able to navigate all the books in the series. Within every chapter, the authors succinctly tell it like they do it. The emphasis is on therapeutic technique; treatment methods are discussed with an eye to appropriate indications, adverse events, and unusual cases. Finally, this book is short and can be read in its entirety on a long plane ride. We believe that brevity paradoxically results in greater information transfer because cover-to-cover mastery is practicable.

Most of the books in the series are accompanied by a high-quality DVD, demonstrating the procedures discussed in that text. Some of you will turn immediately to the DVD and use the text as a backup to clarify complex points, while others will prefer to read first and then view the DVD to see the steps in action. Choose what suits you best.

We hope you enjoy this book and the rest of the books in the series and that you benefit from the many hours of clinical wisdom that have been distilled to produce it. Please keep it nearby, where you can reach for it when you need it.

*Jeffrey S. Dover MD, FRCPC and Murad Alam MD*

To the women in my life

My grandmothers, Bertha and Lillian
My mother, Nina
My daughters, Sophie and Isabel
And especially to my wife, Tania

For their never-ending encouragement, patience, support, love, and friendship

To my father, Mark
A great teacher and role model

To my mentor, Kenneth A. Arndt for his generosity, kindness, sense of humor, joie de vivre, and above all else curiosity and enthusiasm

At Elsevier, Sue Hodgson who conceptualized the series and brought it to reality

and

Martin Mellor for polite, persistent, and dogged determination

*Jeffrey S. Dover*

The professionalism of the dedicated editorial staff at Elsevier has made this ambitious project possible. Guided by the creative vision of Sue Hodgson, Seán Duggan and Martin Mellor have attended to the myriad tasks required to produce a state-of-the-art resource. In this, they have been ably supported by the graphics team, which has maintained production quality while ensuring portability. We are also deeply grateful to the volume editors, who have generously found time in their schedules, cheerfully accepted our guidelines, and recruited the most knowledgeable chapter authors. Finally, we thank the chapter contributors, without whose work there would be no books at all. Whatever successes are herein are due to the efforts of the above, and of my teachers, Kenneth Arndt, Jeffrey Dover, Michael Kaminer, Leonard Goldberg, and David Bickers, and of my parents, Rahat and Rehana Alam.

*Murad Alam*

# Preface

Successful treatment of scars is very difficult. If there were a plethora of good treatments there would be many articles and books about how well these lesions could be improved. But there is little of high quality in the peer reviewed medical literature about this topic, and few if any books published prior to this volume that discuss this dilemma.

Scars come is all sizes, shapes and colors. They may be raised or depressed, thick or thin, ragged or straight, or red white or blue or other hues. They may be very painful or without altered sensation. However they appear and feel and whatever their cause, they are often a reminder of past injury and a focus of current concern, and may as well scar the psyche and soul as well as the skin. With the exception of ritual scarring used as decorative adornments in some cultures, scars are very often a source of misery to patients and of frustration for physicians attempting to improve their appearance or make them disappear.

In this volume there are many excellent contributions from expert authors about all aspects of this topic. After a scholarly discussion of the wound healing process and the formation of scars, there are well written realistic reviews and pragmatic in-depth discussions of the medical, surgical, and radiological approaches to therapy, and the usefulness of lasers and other energy sources for improving scars and altering pigmentation in these lesions. New and innovative approaches are now able to help many patients with unsightly or uncomfortable scars. The pulsed dye laser can bring about very impressive flattening, fading and decreased symptomatology of lesions, topical immune modifiers are being found very useful, new dressings are helpful, and skillful surgical revision and the careful use of ionizing radiation all hold promise of real benefit to the patient with scars. The clever combination concomitant use of several approaches will often bring about the best results. The ability to cover or camouflage cutaneous lesions has become quite sophisticated, and this too is described in detail.

Recent advances in the understanding of connective tissue biology and of wound healing and in treatment strategies and techniques have allowed for much progress in the therapy of scars. It is my hope that the material in this book will be helpful for clinicians who treat scars and for their patients.

*Kenneth A. Arndt, MD*

# List of Contributors


**Christopher J. Ballard** BS
Medical Student, Department of Dermatology and Cutaneous Surgery, University of Miami Miller School of Medicine, Miami, FL, USA

**R. Sonia Batra** MD, MSc, MPH
Section Head, Dermatology and Dermatologic Surgery, City of Hope National Medical Center; Assistant Professor, Beckman Research Institute, Duarte, CA; SkinCare Physicians of Chestnut Hill, Chestnut Hill, MA, USA

**Brian Berman** MD, PhD
Professor, Department of Dermatology and Cutaneous Surgery, University of Miami Miller School of Medicine, Miami, FL, USA

**Joanna Mimi Choi** BA
Medical Student, Harvard Medical School, Boston, MA, USA

**Bahar Dasgeb** MD
Dermatology Fellow, Department of Dermatology, Boston University School of Medicine, Boston, MA, USA

**Roy H. Decker** MD, PhD
Resident Physician, Department of Therapeutic Radiology, Yale University School of Medicine, New Haven, CT, USA

**Galen H Fisher** MD
Mohs and Laser Surgeon, Private Practice, Commonwealth Dermatology, Richmond, VA, USA

**Roy G. Geronemus** MD
Director, Laser & Skin Surgery Center of New York; Clinical Professor, New York University Department of Dermatology, New York, NY, USA

**Michael S. Kaminer** MD
Assistant Professor of Dermatology, Yale Medical School, New Haven, CT and Dartmouth Medical School, Hanover, NH; Director, SkinCare Physicians of Chestnut Hill, Chestnut Hill, MA, USA

**A. Paul Kelly** MD
Professor and Chief, Division of Dermatology, King/Drew Medical Center, Los Angeles, CA, USA

**Keyvan Nouri** MD
Director of Mohs Micrographic, Dermatologic and Laser Surgery; Director of Surgical Training; Associate Professor, Department of Dermatology, Cutaneous Surgery and Otolaryngology, University of Miami Miller School of Medicine, Miami, FL, USA

**Tania J. Phillips** MD, FRCPC
Clinical Professor, Department of Dermatology, Boston University School of Medicine, Boston, MA, USA

**Maria Patricia Rivas** MD
Research Fellow, Department of Dermatology and Cutaneous Surgery, University of Miami, Miami, FL, USA

**Thomas E. Rohrer** MD
Clinical Associate Professor of Dermatology, Boston University School of Medicine; Director of Mohs Fellowship, SkinCare Physicians of Chestnut Hill, Chestnut Hill, MA, USA

**Neil Shear** MD, FRCPC
Head, Department of Dermatology, Sunnybrook Medical Center, Toronto, ON, Canada

**Lynn D. Wilson** MD, MPH
Vice Chairman and Clinical Director; Associate Professor, Department of Therapeutic Radiology, Yale University School of Medicine, New Haven, CT, USA

**Deborah Zell** MD
Clinical Research Fellow, Department of Dermatology and Cutaneous Surgery, University of Miami, FL, USA

# 1 What are Scars?

*Bahar Dasgeb, Tania J. Phillips*

## Introduction

The word **scar** originated from the Greek word **eskhara**, which means scab. It is defined in the Oxford English Dictionary (2004) as a mark left on the skin after healing of a wound or burn. A scar is devoid of skin markings and appendages and may be skin colored, hypo- or hyperpigmented.

A scar reflects the pattern of healing in previously wounded skin. Partial-thickness wounds, which involve epidermis and superficial dermis with preservation of skin appendages, tend to heal without scarring. Full-thickness wounds involve deep dermis and heal with scarring. The spectrum of scarring ranges from minimal to excessive (hypertrophic or keloidal scars).

## Normal Wound Healing

Healing is a dynamic process involving three overlapping phases: (i) inflammation; (ii) granulation tissue formation; and (iii) maturation/remodeling. The relative importance of these steps depends on the depth of tissue loss.

### Partial-thickness wounds

Partial-thickness wounds involve the epidermis and superficial dermis. This results in sparing of the adnexal structures, such as hair follicles, sweat glands, and sebaceous glands. Clot formation, inflammation and granulation tissue formation are minimal. Re-epithelialization, which occurs from the edges of the wound as well as from adnexal structures, is the main step in partial-thickness wound healing. This leads to rapid and complete healing with minimal or no scarring. Pigmentary changes may occur at the wound site.

### Full-thickness wounds

Full-thickness wounds require clot formation to halt bleeding from larger vessels in the deep dermis. Inflammation and granulation are important stages, and contraction is critical in facilitating re-epithelialization by bringing the edges of the wound together. In deep wounds re-epithelialization occurs solely from the epithelial margins due to destruction of adnexal structures. Finally scar tissue is formed to replace the tissue loss.

## Stages of Wound Healing

Knowledge of normal wound healing is important in understanding the pathophysiology of scarring.

### Inflammation

Hematoma formation is the first step in wound healing, and arresting hemorrhage from ruptured vessels as well as proving a temporary barrier to exogenous pathogens. Clot provides a provisional matrix through which inflammatory cell migration occurs. Sequestered platelets degranulate to release a cocktail of growth factors including transforming growth factor beta 1 (TGF-β1), epidermal growth factor (EGF), insulin-like growth factor 1 (IGF-1), and platelet-derived growth factor (PDGF), which initiate signaling pathways leading to recruitment of inflammatory cells, extracellular matrix formation and neovascularization.

A diverse range of other signals such as fibrinolysis by-products serve as chemotactic signals to recruit neutrophils and monocytes to the wound site. These cells migrate from the circulation to the wound by diapedesis through the endothelial lining of capillaries adjacent to the wound site.

The chief role of neutrophils is phagocytosis and intracellular killing of micro-organisms. They also express several pro-inflammatory cytokines that might serve as early signaling pathways to activate local keratinocytes and macrophages. After the acute inflammatory response (24–48 hours), infiltrating monocytes function as activated macrophages, clearing residual pathogens, and cell and matrix debris. These activated macrophages also serve as another source of growth factors and cytokines such as PDGF which stimulate the recruitment of fibroblasts into the site of injury.

### Proliferation

Early granulation tissue is highly vascular and densely cellular. In full-thickness wounds, which do not heal by re-epithelialization alone, dermal fibroblasts adjacent to the wound begin proliferating as an early response. They migrate into the wound, where they lay down an extra-cellular matrix (ECM) composed of fibrin, fibronectin, vitronectin, and glycosaminoglycans (GAG). There is a high ratio of collagen III/collagen I in early granulation tissue. Keratinocytes and fibroblasts start to proliferate in response to growth factors in the wound. As granulation evolves, and an abundant collagen matrix has been deposited, cellularity diminishes due to apoptosis triggered by unknown signals. New blood vessels sprout into the extracellular matrix triggered by angiogenesis molecules, inducing vascular endothelial growth factor (VEGF), TGF-β1, angiotropin, and thrombospondin. In large wounds, contraction mediated by transformed wound fibroblasts (myofibroblasts) reduces the quantity of granulation tissue needed to fill the defect and minimizes the area of re-epithelialization needed to replace tissue loss. Fibroblasts also provide wound edge tension through contractile proteins actin and desmin. The release of mechanical tension after the wound has closed sends 'stop' signals for wound contraction. Re-epithelialization of wounds begins hours after injury. Migrating keratinocytes up-grade tissue-type and urokinase-type plasminogen activators (tPA and uPA) and receptors for uPA to activate fibrinolysis, an essential step for keratinocyte migration.

In order to crawl over the provisional matrix keratinocytes express new receptors for fibronectin and collagen. Keratinocyte migration and re-epithelialization is facilitated by wound contraction.

### Remodeling

During the remodeling phase of healing, excess collagen and matrix are removed by tissue enzymes, and inflammatory cells leave the wound. Scar maturation involves a balance of matrix degradation and collagen biosynthesis. While fibroblasts synthesize collagen, contractile proteins and extracellular matrix, a variety of enzymes (matrix metalloproteinases) involved in degradation and remodeling are released by fibroblasts, mast cells, endothelial cells, and macrophages. The balance between these proteinases and their inhibitors (TIMP I and TIMP II) play an important role in tissue repair. Interferons produced by T lymphocytes (interferon-gamma), leucocytes (interferon-alpha) and fibroblasts (interferon-beta) have antifibrotic activity and inhibit fibroblast synthesis of collagen and fibronectin. The remodeling process occurs over 6–12 months but can persist for years after the initial injury. Scar strength usually achieves 70–80% of the tensile strength of normal skin and scar tissue is therefore more vulnerable to re-injury.

## Types of Scarring

### Normal scars

Any injury that extends into the dermis will always heal with a scar. Early scars are formed in 7–10 days after injury and have a high ratio of collagen III/collagen I; they only demonstrate 5–10% of the skin's original breaking strength. Over the next 6–12 months, the wound undergoes significant remodeling, characterized by collagen deposition and cross-linking, resulting in the establishment of a mature scar, mainly replaced by type I collagen and approximating 80% of the original tissue strength.

### Abnormal scars

Cutaneous wounds sometimes heal with exuberant scarring to form hypertrophic scars or keloid scars. The basis for abnormal scarring has not been fully elucidated, but it is known that hypertrophic scars and keloids depart early from the normal wound healing process and rarely involute spontaneously. The formation of new collagen following the inflammatory stage extends over a much longer period of time than in normal healing. Collagen synthesis is significantly (approximately 20 times) higher than in normal skin, with increased turnover, resulting in a disproportionate amount of collagen deposition.

Fibroblasts from keloid scars produce increased amounts of collagen per cell, in vitro as well as in vivo, even in the absence of growth factors. Elevated levels of collagenase, as well as collagenase inhibitors, have been found in keloids.

Altered levels of immunoregulatory cytokines may play a role in keloid formation: patients with keloids were found to have higher levels of interleukin 6, TNF-alpha and interferon-beta than normal controls. The production of interferon-alpha, interferon-gamma and TNF-beta were markedly depressed in keloid patients. Keloid formation has been postulated to be due not only to a fibroblast defect but also in keratinocyte control over the fibroblast. Keloid-derived human keratinocytes (KHKs) induce increased proliferation in normal dermal human fibroblasts (NHFs) compared to normal human keratinocytes, and induce NHFs to secrete collagen in a pattern similar to keloid tissue. Keloid-derived human fibroblasts co-cultured with KHKs showed even higher proliferation rates, indicating an intrinsic abnormality of both keratinocytes and fibroblasts.

Growth factors such as insulin-like growth factor may play an important role in the regulation of KHF proliferation in co-culture with KHKs.

## TGF-beta

TGF-beta has emerged as a likely candidate for inducing excess scar and keloid formation. TGF-beta induces fibroblast collagen, fibronectin and proteoglycan synthesis. It also decreases collagenase production and increases production of collagenase inhibitors, thus reducing matrix degradation. Three isoforms of TGF-beta (1, 2, and 3) have been identified in mammals. Keloid fibroblasts are particularly sensitive to isoforms of TGF-β1 and TGF-β2, which have pro-fibrotic functions and increase scar formation.

In a controlled study, wound treatment with neutralizing antibodies to TGF-β1 and -β2 reduced collagen deposition and scarring compared to control wounds in rodents. Addition of TGF-β3 reduced the monocyte and macrophage profile, inflammation, fibronectin, and collagen I and III deposition in early stages of wound healing, improved the architecture of the neodermis, and reduced scarring. It has been reported that TGF-β3 isoforms increased in intensity from day 7 post wounding in old mice, while TGF-β1 and -β2 isoforms were increased at all time points in the wounds of younger mice. This could explain to some degree the improved quality of tissue repair and decreased quantity of scar formation in the older population. The relative proportion of TGF-β isoforms, such as the ratio of TGF-β3 to TGF-β1 may determine the wound repair outcome.

## Matrix metalloproteinases

Matrix metalloproteinases (MMPs) are tissue enzymes which play a major role in remodeling of ECM during wound healing. The composition of the extracellular matrix in fetal skin and wounds differs from that in adults. It has been suggested that differential expression of MMPs and TIMPs occurs during the ontogenetic transition to scar-forming wound repair.

Expression of MMPs and TIMPs appears to be carefully regulated during normal wound healing. An imbalance between MMPs and TIMPs activity can impair wound healing and cause abnormal scar formation. MMP1 is significantly upregulated in both scarless and scarring wounds. However the maximal increase in expression of MMP1 and MMP9 occurred more rapidly and was much greater in scarless fetal wounds.

While unchanged in scarless wounds, MMP2 levels decreased more than 3-fold in scarring wounds. Levels of MMP1 and MMP3 were increased in scar-forming wounds. Overall it appeared that scarless wound repair is associated with a higher ratio of MMP to TIMP expression compared to scarring wounds.

## Apoptosis

Apoptosis, also called **programmed cell death**, is genetically determined and necessary for maintaining tissue homeostasis. Apoptosis is modulated by several intrinsic and extrinsic signals. In normal wound healing, apoptosis is thought to play a role in the transition from granulation tissue into definitive scar tissue. In this transition period, several cells types including fibroblasts, inflammatory cells, endothelial cells, and possibly most importantly myofibroblasts, undergo apoptosis.

Keloid fibroblasts have been shown to have lower rates of apoptosis than normal skin fibroblasts. Several mechanisms have been suggested as responsible for this resistance to apoptosis observed in keloidal tissue; these will be discussed in turn. Table 1.1 summarizes the pro-apoptotic/anti-apoptotic effects of the genes and proteins which are described in this chapter.

The *p53* gene has been implicated in having tumor-suppression functions by controlling cell proliferation and apoptosis; moreover mutations of this gene are associated to a variety of sporadic human tumors. Saed et al identified *p53* gene focal mutations in keloidal fibroblasts by polymerase chain reaction (PCR), single-strand conformational polymorphism (SSCP) and confirmed by DNA sequencing. No mutations were observed in fibroblasts from normal skin of the same patients.

In a different study, a dysregulation of *p53* and upregulation of *bcl-2* was found in the younger, hypercellular peripheral areas of the keloid along with a lower rate of apoptosis compared to controls. In contrast, Fas expression was observed to be more prominent in the central, hypocellular regions of the keloids. TGF-β1 is thought to be responsible for the resistance to apoptosis observed in keloid-derived fibroblasts,

| Apoptotic Function | |
|---|---|
| **Pro-apoptotic** | **Anti-apoptotic** |
| Caspase 3 | Bcl |
| Caspase 6 | DAD-1 |
| Caspase 8 | ERK |
| c-myc | GST |
| NIP-3 | GSTM |
| HDLC-1 | GP |
| TRADD | JNK |
| TNF* | TNF* |

**TNF can induce both cell death and cell survival.*

**Table 1.1** Apoptotic Function

as the expression of Fas-mediated apoptosis was not decreased in keloidal fibroblasts as compared to hypertrophic scar-derived and normal skin-derived fibroblasts when TGF-β1 was added. Keloid fibroblasts have also been shown to resist apoptosis induced by ceramide, which is believed to be mediated by increased levels of insulin growth factor (IGF).

Two major groups of genes for apoptosis that appear to have a role in keloid biology were identified by Woolery-Lloyd and Berman. They include the caspase family and the TNF family. The caspase family is a group of pro-apoptotic proteases in which sequential activation of one caspase by another leads to a cascade of proteolytic activity and cell death. Caspase-8, -13, and 14 were found to be upregulated in keloids when compared to adjacent normal skin. Caspase-8 is the first enzyme in the cascade activated by the binding of the Fas and TNF receptor. Caspase-13 is also a pro-apoptotic enzyme which is activated by caspase-8. Interestingly, caspase-14 is not known to participate in a pro-apoptotic pathway and is only expressed in keratinocytes. Caspase-6, a pro-apoptotic protein, was found to be downregulated in keloids. The TNF superfamily includes both the TNF ligand and the TNF receptor family. Compared to normal skin, TNFSF12 and TNFSF14 (ligands) were upregulated, whereas TNFRSF10B and TNFRSF1B (receptors) were downregulated. Interestingly, fibroblasts from keloids had lower expression of apoptotic genes, primarily from the caspase and TNF superfamily, in the presence of TNF-alpha, when compared to normal fibroblasts. This resistance to apoptosis could be explained by the decreased number of TNF receptors on keloidal fibroblasts.

Sayah and colleagues compared the expression of 64 apoptosis-related genes in keloids and normal scars. Eight of 64 genes were found to be significantly (difference >50%) underexpressed in keloidal tissue: TRADD, *c-myc* protooncogene, NIP-3, HDLC-1, which are promoters of apoptosis and DAD-1, G-S-T, G-S-T-M, and glutathione peroxidase, which are apoptosis inhibitors.

Epidermal keratinocytes have been implicated to play a role in dermal fibroblast regulation. Keloidal fibroblasts cultured with keloid-derived keratinocytes proliferated more than those cultured with normal skin keratinocytes. Moreover, keloidal fibroblast cultures with keloidal keratinocytes are more resistant to apoptosis than normal ones cultured with normal skin keratinocytes. Decreased levels of caspase-3, a pro-apoptotic factor, and increased expression of bcl-2 and increased ERK and JNK phosphorylation, all anti-apoptotic factors, were found in keloidal fibroblasts cultured with keloidal keratinocytes. These data and the fact that caspase-14, which is only know to be expressed in keratinocytes, was upregulated in keloids suggests that there may be an interaction between the epidermis and dermis in keloid biology.

Dysregulation of the expression of genes associated with apoptosis may allow fibroblasts to undergo apoptosis at a lower rate and continue to produce and secrete extracellular matrix beyond the time expected in normal scarring, which explains the progressive nature of keloids. Apoptosis may have a role in two distinctive times of wound healing.

The first implicates the downregulation of inflammatory cell infiltration that occurs between the inflammatory and proliferative phases, therefore those factors that are anti-apoptotic, will allow inflammatory cells to stay longer, having a profibrotic effect. The second possible role of apoptosis implicates the downregulation of fibroblasts and its product collagen, where anti-apoptotic factors will increase collagen deposition; this is observed in keloidal scarring.

The University of Connecticut Health Center is currently conducting a study to determine the pivotal gene implicated in setting up the fibrotic response in keloids, by performing genome-wide screening and linkage analysis in families with subjects with and without keloidal disease.

In conclusion, there are several genes that appear to play a significant role in keloid biology. It is believed that the greater proliferative capacity observed in keloidal fibroblasts might be due not only to an increased proliferation rate, but also to lower rates of apoptosis. It remains unclear how these genes interact and the exact role they play in keloid pathogenesis, however it is clear that in keloids, apoptosis regulation is different. Further studies are needed to explain the role of programmed cell death in keloids, as this may provide a target for prevention and treatment of this condition (Fig. 1.1).

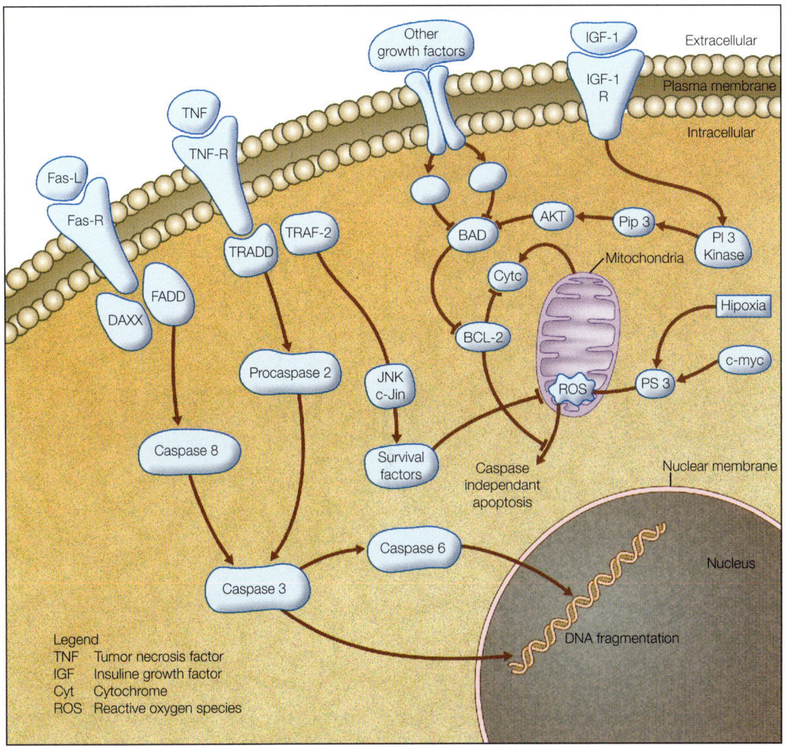


**Fig. 1.1** Apoptotic signals with projected mechanisms of action in keloid pathways. Cyt = cytochrome, IGF = insulin growth factor, ROS = reactive oxygen species, TNF = tumor necrosis factor. Other nonillustrated mediators = ceramide, caspase 13, caspase 14, NIP-3, HDLC-1, DAD-1, G-S-T, G-S-T-M, ERK, GP

## Clinical and Pathologic Features of Scars

### Hypertrophic scars

Hypertrophic scars (Table 1.2) are confined to the boundary of the original injury and increase in bulk by pushing out the margin, rather than invasion. They are usually asymptomatic, develop within weeks after the injury and tend to gradually resolve. They are common among younger individuals. They may develop hypo- or hyperpigmentation over time and tend to have a smooth surface. Hypertrophic scars (Fig. 1.2) and keloids share some clinical features. For example, the overlying epidermis in hypertrophic scars and keloid scars is thin and lacks normal skin markings and appendages. Common sites include the earlobe, upper chest, upper back, and deltoid region. They are rare on the mucous membranes, palms, soles, penis, scrotum and eyelids.

#### *Histopathology*

Hypertrophic scars are characterized by fibrillary collagen arranged parallel to the skin surface, with an increased number of fibroblasts having the same alignment (Fig. 1.3).

Hypertrophic scars contain myofibroblasts, which are not found in keloid scars. Elastin, which is abundantly present in normal skin and normal scars, is rarely found in hypertrophic scars or keloids. Blood vessels are prominent with a vertical arrangement perpendicular to the

| Key Features of Normal, Hypertrophic, and Keloid Scars | | |
|---|---|---|
| **Normal scars** | **Hypertrophic scars** | **Keloid scars** |
| Develop after days 7–10 | Develop in weeks | Develop in months |
| Any age | Young individuals | Any age – peak age: 10–30 |
| Asymptomatic | Familial inheritance | Familial inheritance |
| Nonvascular | Asymptomatic | Tender, pruritic |
| Within the wound border | Highly vascular | Highly vascular |
| Flat | Within the wound border | Extends beyond the wound border |
| Contraction | Raised | Raised |
| Spontaneous resolution | Contraction | No contraction |
| Hypo-/hyperpigmented | May resolve<br>Red, or hypo-/hyperpigmented | Rarely resolve<br>Red, or hypo-/hyperpigmented |

**Table 1.2** Key features of normal, hypertrophic, and keloid scars

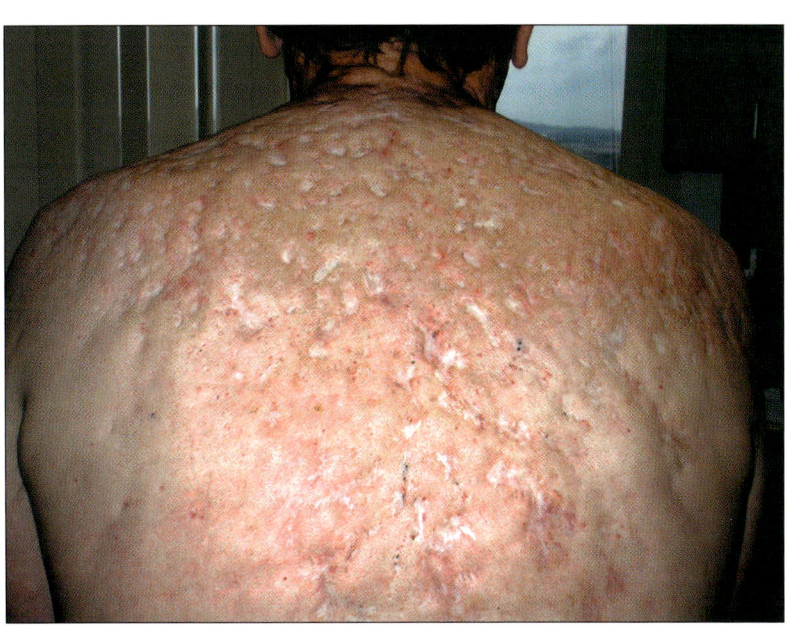

**Fig. 1.2** Hypertrophic and atrophic scars, late stage

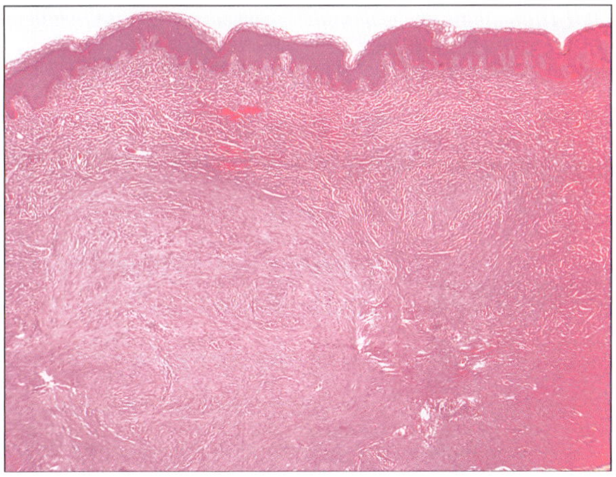

**Fig. 1.3** Histopathologic features of hypertrophic scars. There is a large nodular, paucicellular area of fibrosis with vertically oriented blood vessels. Note that the epidermis is not flattened in this case. (Courtesy of Dr Samer Ghosn, Boston University School of Medicine)

skin surface. Electron microscopy has shown partially or totally occluded blood vessels in both hypertrophic scars and keloids.

## Keloid scars

Keloids, from the Greek word **chele**, or **crab claw** are irregularly shaped scars which extend beyond the borders of the original wound. Unlike hypertrophic scars, keloids tend to persist over time. They are usually broad nodular scars, and tend to have a rope-like surface. They extend into adjacent tissue and are often symptomatic, associated with pruritus and tenderness. They occur in all skin types, but individuals with darkly pigmented skin have a higher risk for keloid formation (Fig. 1.4), with an incidence of up to 16% in the black population.

Keloids are unusual in infants and the elderly, with a peak incidence between the ages of 10 and 30. The male:female ratio is approximately 1:1. Although a family tendency is reported, there is no clear inheritance pattern.

## *Histopathology*

Collagen bundles in keloids are distinctively thickened and eosinophilic, and arranged in nodular arrays. Fibroblasts in keloid scars have plumper nuclei that those seen in other scars. Keloids are highly vascular with excessive endothelial cell proliferation that can sometimes causes vessel occlusion and may develop calcification.

Triggers for excess inflammation, such as infection, excessive wound tension, and foreign material are implicated in the keloid response. It has been reported that keloids, transplanted to areas of low tension, have subsequently resolved.

Melanocytes may play a role since keloids have not been reported in albinos and occur more often in darkly pigmented individuals. Mast cells, whose mediators are known to upregulate collagen synthesis, are numerous in both hypertrophic scars and keloids (Fig. 1.5) compared with normal scars and uninjured skin.

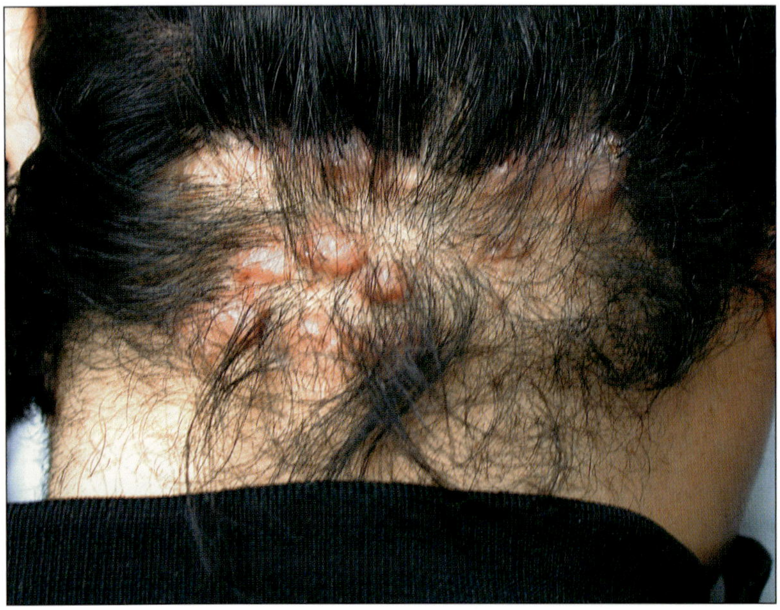

**Fig. 1.4** Keloids

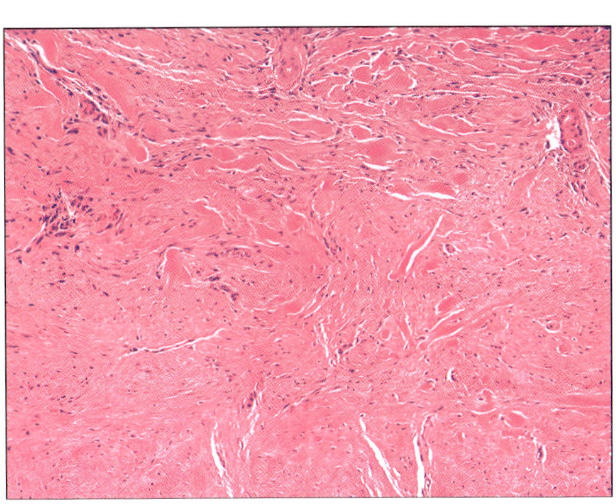

**Fig. 1.5** Histopathologic features of keloids. Note the broad homogeneous eosinophilic keloidal collagen that contrasts with the surrounding fibrotic tissue. (Courtesy of Dr Samer Ghosn, Boston University School of Medicine)

### Atrophic scars

These scars are more common than hypertrophic scars or keloids. Atrophic scars are thin and wrinkled. They are occasionally depressed and may resemble primary atrophy.

These scars are confined to the boundaries of injured skin and lie below the surface of the uninjured surrounding skin. They occur independently of age, are usually asymptomatic, and can develop at any site.

#### *Histopathology*

The collagen pattern in atrophic scars resembles that of hypertrophic scars. Atrophic scars are significantly less vascular and cellular.

The histopathologic features of hypertrophic scars and keloids are summarized in Table 1.3.

## Factors that Influence Scarring

### Age

#### *Scarless fetal wound healing*

It has been observed that skin wound healing in the fetus is very different to the process in adults: it occurs rapidly and scarlessly. The mechanisms that underlie scarless fetal tissue repair are unknown, but it is known that wound healing occurs with very little inflammation, there are large amounts of hyaluronic acid deposited in the wound matrix, and collagen is deposited in an organized manner.

The fetal wound environment differs from the adult's in many ways. The fetus is relatively hypoxemic, and fetal tissue oxygenation remains low throughout gestation.

| Histopathologic Features of Hypertrophic and Keloid Scars | | |
|---|---|---|
| **Normal scar** | **Hypertrophic scar** | **Keloid scars** |
| Thin, wavy collagen bundles parallel to skin surface, Elastin present | Fibrillary collagen bundles parallel to skin surface Elastin usually absent | Thickened eosinophilic collagen bands Nodules in concentric arrangement Elastin usually absent |
| Noncellular | Myofibroblasts are present Fibroblasts have normal nuclei, aligned parallel to skin surface Mast calls and plasma cells present | Myofibroblasts are absent Increased number of fibroblast with big nuclei, in no regular order Mast cell and plasma cells present |
| Nonvascular | Prominent blood vessels (perpendicular to skin surface) Endothelial hypertrophy and occasional vascular occlusion | Highly vascular (perpendicular to skin surface) Endothelial hypertrophy and predominant vascular occlusion |
| No calcification | No calcification | Calcification may be present |
| Flattened epidermis | Flattened epidermis | Nonflattened epidermis |
| Fibrotic papillary dermis | Fibrotic papillary dermis | Nonfibrotic papillary dermis |
| No advancing edge | No advancing edge | Tongue-like advancing edge – underneath normal-appearing epidermis + dermis |

**Table 1.3** Histopathologic features of hypertrophic and keloid scars

There is minimal inflammatory response to fetal skin injury due to lack of neutrophils in the wound matrix. As the immune system develops later in gestation and its resultant inflammatory response increases, scar formation occurs at the repair site.

Fetal skin wounds are continually bathed in warm, sterile amniotic fluid, known to be rich in growth factors. However amniotic fluid is not critical for scarless healing. Fetal lamb studies have shown that exclusion of wounds from amniotic fluid by a Silastic patch does not prevent scarless repair, and that adult skin transplanted to the fetus heals with scar formation despite exposure to amniotic fluid.

The hyaluronic acid-rich ECM environment facilitates cell mobility, cell proliferation, and repair of fetal wounds, and is likely the most important factor in scarless healing. The prolonged presence of a glycoprotein called hyaluronic-acid-stimulating activity (HASA) in fetal wounds, which is entirely absent in adult wounds, may facilitate the orderly deposition of collagen. Experimental tympanic membrane perforations in rats treated with hyaluronic acid (HA) not only close faster than in untreated controls, but also show much less scar tissue, with a discernible organized collagen fiber layer.

Rapid epithelialization in fetal wounds may be related to deposition of fibronectin and tenascin early in the fetal wound matrix. There are phenotypic differences between adult and fetal fibroblasts. Early fetal fibroblasts synthesize more type III and IV collagen compared to adult counterparts that mainly produce collagen type I. Fetal fibroblasts are also capable of proliferating simultaneously while synthesizing collagen, while in adults proliferation needs to occur first before fibroblasts are ready to lay down collagen. As a result, collagen deposition is delayed in adult wound healing, leading to scar formation. Contraction has almost no role in scarless repair, because fetal wounds have virtually no myofibroblasts.

Inflammation plays a key role in tissue repair and scar formation. In the absence of inflammation, embryos are able to heal wounds without scarring. There is a general consensus that wound healing is impaired with aging. Aging appears to diminish inflammatory responses with impaired macrophage and T-cell function, loss of fibroblast responsiveness and motility, as well as reduced quantity and distribution pattern of various growth factors and their receptors including TGF-beta. This might explain age-related differences seen in wound healing speed and quality. Although the rate of wound healing is impaired in the elderly, the quality of scarring is improved. This may be related to reduced TGF-beta levels in wounded skin. It is also possible that in wounds in the elderly, a subpopulation of fibroblasts with a fetal phenotype is present, which results in a fetal wound healing-like response. Hormones, such as estrogen, which decline after menopause, may also play a role in delayed wound closure and decreased scarring in aging individuals.

## Genetics

There is frequently a family history of keloids and the incidence is much higher in pigmented skin, ranging from 4.5–16% in the black and Hispanic populations. Both autosomal dominant and recessive patterns of inheritance have been reported.

There is a higher incidence of keloids in patients with HLA-β14, BW16, blood group A, and in Rubenstein-Taybi syndrome.

## Hormones: estrogen

In vitro studies have shown that reproductive hormones influence certain pivotal steps in wound healing, such as proliferation and inflammation. Estrogen may regulate the production of TGF-beta isoforms and their receptors, which play a significant role in fibrosis and scar formation. Aging in healthy females is associated with a reduced rate of cutaneous wound healing, but an improved quality of scarring, with reduced levels of TGF-β1 in the wound. Hormone replacement therapy can reverse delayed wound repair in postmenopausal females, suggesting that wound healing is modulated either directly or indirectly by circulating reproductive hormones. Studies in humans have shown that systemic hormone replacement therapy for 3 months can accelerate re-epithelialization and collagen deposition of acute wounds in postmenopausal females.

The presence of estrogen receptors on fibroblasts suggests that estrogen may directly modulate the function of these cells. Estrogen has been shown to increase the levels of TGF-β1 in vitro.

These data suggest that estrogen is involved in dermal fibroblast production and/or secretion of TGF-β1. Finally it is interesting that systemic estrogen antagonists can reduce scarring in humans. Preliminary analysis of scars from women wounded while taking the estrogen antagonist tamoxifen show these are of superior quality compared with scars from equivalent wounds in women not treated with tamoxifen.

## Summary

Scars occur after healing of full-thickness wounds. Pathologic hypertrophic, or keloidal scars can present difficult management problems. While some progress has been made in understanding the pathophysiology of abnormal scarring, there is still a great deal to be learned before targeted therapeutic strategies can be optimized.

## Acknowledgment

The authors would like to thank Brian Berman and Claudia C. Ramirez for the section on Apoptosis.

### Further Reading

Adzick S, Longaker M 1992 Scarless fetal healing. Annals of Surgery 215:3–7
Ashcroft G, Dodsworth J, Boxtel E, et al 1997 Estrogen accelerates cutaneous wound healing associated with an increase in TGF-beta 1 level. Nature Medicine 3:1209–1215
Ashcroft G, Horan M, Ferguson M 1997 The effect of aging on wound healing: Immunolocalization of growth factors and their receptors in a murine incisional model. Journal of Anatomy 190:351–365
Bloom D 1956 Heredity of keloids: A review of the literature and a report of a family with multiple keloids in 5 generations. New York State Medicine 56:511–519
Burton C 2003 Dermal hypertrophies. In: Bolognia J, Jorizzo J, Rapini R (eds) Dermatology. Mosby, London, pp 1531–1537
Calnan J, Copenhagen H 1967 Auto-transplantation of keloid in men. British Journal of Surgery 54:330–335
Carlson MA, Longaker MT 2004 The fibroblast-populated collagen matrix as a model of wound healing: a review of the evidence. Wound Repair and Regeneration 12:134–147
Castagnoli C, Perveci OD, Stella AA, et al 1990 The HLA B-16 allogenotype constitutes a risk factor for hypertrophic scarring. Human Immunology 24:229–232
Chodon T, Sugihara T, Igawa HH, Funayama E, Furukawa H 2000 Keloid-derived fibroblasts are refractory to Fas-mediated apoptosis and neutralization of autocrine transforming growth factor-beta1 can abrogate this resistance. American Journal of Pathology 157:1661–1669
Clark RAF 1996 Wound repair: Overview and general consideration. In: Clark RAF (ed.) The Molecular and Cellular Biology of Wound Repair. New York, Plenum Press, pp 3–50
Cohen IK, Keiser HR, Sjoerdgmo A 1971 Collagen synthesis in human keloid & hypertrophic scar. Surgical Forum 22:488
Dang C, Beanes S, Lee H, Zhang X, Soo C, Ting K 2003 Scarless fetal wounds are associated with an increase matrix metalloproteinase-to-tissue-derived inhibitor of metalloproteinase ratio. Plastic and Reconstructive Surgery 111:2273–2285
Desmouliere A, Redard M, Darby I, Gabbiani G 1995 Apoptosis mediates the decrease in cellularity during the transition between granulation tissue and scar. American Journal of Pathology 146:56–66
Diegelman RF, Bryant CP, Cohen IK 1977 Tissue alpha globulins in keloid formation. Plastic and Reconstructive Surgery 59:418–423
Diegelman RF, Cohen IK, McCoy B 1979 Growth kinetics and collagen synthesis of normal skin scar and keloidal fibroblasts in vitro. Journal of Cell Physiology 98:341–346
Estes JM, Vande Berg JS, Adzick NS, MacGillivray TE, Desmouliere A, Gabbiani G 1994 Phenotypic and functional features of myofibroblasts in sheep fetal wounds. Differentiation 56:173–181

Fitzpatrick T, Bernhard J, Cropley T 1999 The structures of skin lesions and fundamentals of diagnosis. In: Freedberg IM, Eisen AZ, Wolff K et al (eds) Fitzpatrick's Dermatology in General Medicine. 5th edn. McGraw Hill, New York, pp 29, P1163–P1165
Funayama E, Chodon T, Oyama A, Sugihara T 2003 Keratinocytes promote proliferation and inhibit apoptosis of the underlying fibroblasts: an important role in the pathogenesis of keloid. Journal of Investigative Dermatology 121(6):1326–1331
Grondahl HJ, Lund LR, Ralfkiaer E, et al 1988 Urokinase and tissue plasminogen activators in keratinocytes during wound reepithelialization in vivo. Journal of Investigative Dermatology 90:790–795
He Y, Grinnell F 1994 Stress relaxation of fibroblasts activates a cyclic AMP signaling pathway. Journal of Cell Biology 126:457–464
Hubner G, Brauchle M, Smola H, et al 1996 Differential regulation of pro-inflammatory cytokines during wound healing in normal and glucocorticoid treated mice. Cytokine 8:548–556
Humke EW, Ni J, Dixit VM 1998 ERICE, a novel FLICE-activatable caspase. Journal of Biological Chemistry 273:15702–15707
Ishihara H, Yoshimoto H, Fujioka M, et al 2000 Keloid fibroblasts resist ceramide-induced apoptosis by overexpression of insulin-like growth factor I receptor. Journal of Investigative Dermatology 115:1065–1071
Kalvakolanu DV, Bradon EC 1996 An overview of the interferon system: Signal transduction & mechanisms of action. Cancer Investigation 14:25
Kim IJ, Phan TT, Song C, Wan WT, Longaker AK 2001 Investigation of the influence of keloid-derived keratinocytes on fibroblast growth and proliferation in vitro. Plastic and Reconstructive Surgery 107:797–808
Kirsner CW 1992 The microvessels in hypertrophic scars, keloidal scars and related lesions: A review. Journal of Submicroscopic Cytology and Pathology 24:281–296
Kurwa AR 1979 Rubenstein – Taybi syndrome and spontaneous keloids. Clinical and Experimental Dermatology 4:251
Ladin DA, Hou Z, Patel D, et al 1998 p53 and apoptosis alterations in keloids and keloid fibroblasts. Wound Repair and Regeneration 6:28–37
Lawrentaci G, Diguardi D 1977 HLA antigen in keloids and hypertrophic scars. Archives of Dermatology 113:1726
Lee JY, Yang CC, Chao SC, Wong TW 2004 Histopathology diagnosis of keloid and hypertrophic scars. American Journal of Dermatopathology 26:379
Lever W 1983 Tumors of fibrous tissue. In: Lever WF (ed) Histopathology of the Skin. 6th edn. Lippincott, Philadelphia, pp 604–606
Linares HA, Larson DL 1978 Proteoglycans and collagenases in hypertrophic scar formation. Plastic and Reconstructive Surgery 62:589–593
Longaker M, Burd DAR, Yen TSB, et al 1991 Midgestation fetal lamb excisional wound contact in utero. Journal of Pediatric Surgery 26:942–948
Longaker MT, Whitby DJ, Crombleholme TM, et al 1989 Studies in fetal wound healing III. Early deposition of adhesion molecules distinguishes fetal from adult wounds. Journal of Pediatric Surgery 24:789–804
Longaker M, Whitby D, Jennings R, et al 1990 Adult skin in the fetal environment heals with scar formation. Surgical Forum 41:639–641
McCauley RL, Chopra V, Li YY, Herndon DN, Robson MC 1992 Altered cytokine production in black patients with keloids. Journal of Clinical Immunolog 12:300–308
Mehendale F, Martin P 2001 The cellular and molecular events of wound healing. In: Falanga V (ed.) Cutaneous Wound Healing. Martin Dunitz, London, pp 15–36
Messadi DV, Le A, Berg S, et al 1999 Expression of apoptosis-associated genes by human dermal scar fibroblasts. Wound Repair and Regeneration 7:511–517
Murray JC, Pollack SV, Pinnell SR 1981 Keloids: A review. Journal of the American Academy of Dermatology 4:461–470
Nelson N 1976 Respiration and circulation before birth. In: Smith CA, N. Nelson (eds) The Physiology of the Newborn Infant. 4th edn. Charles Thomas, Springfield, IL, pp 15–17
Peacock EE, Madden JW, Trier WC 1970 Biologic basis for the treatment of keloids and hypertrophic scars. South African Medical Journal 1970;63;755–760
Peled ZM, Phelps ED, Updike DL, et al 2002 Matrix metalloproteinases and the ontogeny of scarless repair: the other side of the wound healing balance. Plastic and Reconstructive Surgery 110:801–811
Phillips T 1999 Aging and wound healing. Wounds 11(Suppl):2D–6D
Romer J, Lund LR, Eriksen J, et al 1991 Differential expression of urokinase-type plasminogen activator and its type-1 inhibitor during healing of mouse skin wound. Investigative Dermatology 1991;97:803–811
Romer J, Lund LR, Eriksen J, et al 1994 The receptor for urokinase plasminogen activator is expressed by keratinocytes at the leading edge during reepithelialization of mouse skin wound. Journal of Investigative Dermatology 102:519–522
Saed G, Ladin D, Olson J, Han X, Fivenson D 1997 p53 and apoptosis in the pathogenesis of keloids [abstract]. Journal of Investigative Dermatology 108:A580

Saed GM, Ladin D, Olson J, Han X, Hou Z, Fivenson D 1998 Analysis of p53 gene mutations in keloids using polymerase chain reaction-based single-strand conformational polymorphism and DNA sequencing. Archives of Dermatology 134:963–967

Sayah DN, Soo C, Shaw WW, et al 1999 Downregulation of apoptosis-related genes in keloid tissues. Surgical Research 87:209–216

Shah M, Foreman DM, Ferguson MW 1994 Neutralizing antibody to TGFBeta 1, 2 reduces scarring in adult rodents. Journal of Cell Science 107:1137–1157

Simpson D, Ross R 1972 The neutrophilic leukocytes in wound repair; a study with anti-neutrophilic serum. Journal of Clinical Investigation 51:2009–2023

Singer AJ, Clarke RAF 1999 Cutaneous wound healing. New England Journal of Medicine 341:738–746

Thomas B, Krummel T, Melang M, et al 1988 Collagen synthesis and type expression by fetal fibroblast in vitro. Surgical Forum 39:642–643

Thompson CB 1995 Apoptosis in the pathogenesis and treatment of disease. Science 267:1456–1462

Urioste SS, Arndt KA, Dover JS 1999 Keloids and hypertrophic scars: review and treatment strategies. Seminars in Cutaneous Medicine and Surgery 18:159–171

White C, Barnhill R 2004 Collagen and elastin. In: White C, Barnhill R (eds) Text book of Dermatopathology. 2nd edn. McGraw Hill, New York, pp 405–426

W-Lloyd H, Berman B, Vincek V, Nassiri M 2003 A comparison of expression of apoptotic markers in keloids and control skin. Presented at the Residents and Fellows symposium, American Academy Dermatology, 2003

Yang GP, Lim IJ, Phan TT, Lorenz HP, Longaker AK 2003 From scarless fetal wounds to keloids: Molecular studies in wound healing. Wound Repair and Regeneration 11:411–418

# 2 Medical Treatment of Scarring

*Brian Berman, Deborah Zell*

## Introduction

Scars are the visible and tactile changes following the healing process of an injury. Excessive scarring can be the result of atypical wound healing and have excess dense fibrous tissue deposited haphazardly forming either hypertrophic scars or keloids. Hypertrophic scars are generally red and raised, and remain within the boundaries of the original site of injury. Keloids are scars that extend beyond the site of the original wound, taking sometimes years to appear after the original injury.

Histologically, both keloids and hypertrophic scars have a high density of fibroblasts and collagen fibrils, rich vasculature, and thickened epidermal cell layers. The two conditions differ histologically in that hypertrophic scars generally have more parallel, flat bundles of organized collagen sheets than do keloids, which characteristically have disarrayed collagen sheets.

Scars can be solitary, multiple, localized, widespread, elevated, depressed, hyperpigmented, hypopigmented, and/or contracted. In order to help assess the type of treatment needed for each individual scar the following should be considered: the inciting cause, anatomic location, relaxed skin tension lines (RSTLs), and the type of scar (hypertrophic, atrophic, keloidal [Fig. 2.1]). Therefore, each scar and its treatment require evaluation on an individual basis.

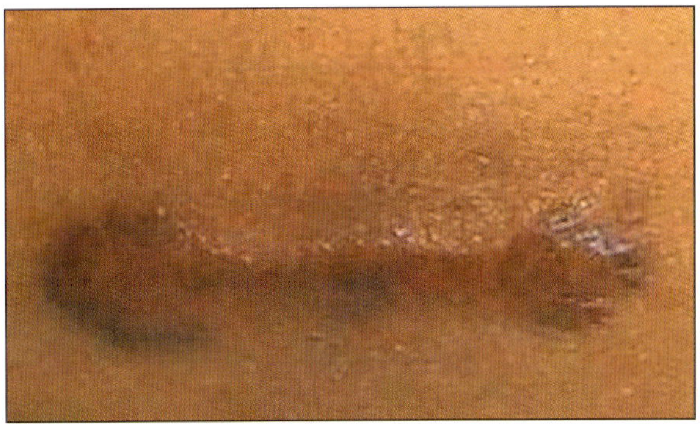

**Fig. 2.1** Keloids. A dark-skinned individual status post treatment with occlusion therapy to the central portion of the keloid. TNF = tumor necrosis factor, IGF = insulin growth factor, cyt = cytochrome, ROS = reactive oxygen species

The type of scar, location, symptoms, and psychological readiness of the patient to desire a change should all be acknowledged when considering treatment of a scar. Most scars and hypertrophic scars are mainly cosmetic concerns. Keloids can also be painful, tender and pruritic. Scars can cause a loss of function (contracture overlying a joint), as well as significant disfigurement. The psychological trauma of scars can be an emotionally charged subject for patients. They may require counseling or psychological help and a possible waiting period for dealing with these sensitive issues before treatment can take place, since the patient may need time to logically think about the physician's treatment plans for the scar.

It is important for patients to realize that the medical elimination of scars is nearly impossible. Improvement can be made although the scar may only become smaller, less pigmented, flatter, or less noticeable. Cosmetically favorable scars are fine, flat, well positioned, and are located at the periphery of the face, at a transition between two cosmetic subunits, or at a midline position. On the other hand, unsightly scars lack these qualities and are made more noticeable by pigmentation, elevation, anatomical location or position (overlying two cosmetic areas).

Scar location and orientation are important for cosmetically favorable scars (Table 2.1), and the RSTLs are used as a guide to help make scars less noticeable. The RSTLs determine the directional tendency and elastic properties of the skin. The formation of the RSTLs is

| Cosmetically Favorable and Unfavorable Scars | | |
|---|---|---|
| **Category** | **Favorable scars** | **Unfavorable scars** |
| Location | Between two cosmetic subunits or directly midline | Lie in two cosmetic subunits |
| Configuration | Parallel to RSTLs | Perpendicular to RSTLs |
| Depth | Shallow | Deep |
| Color | Skin colored | Hyperpigmented or hypopigmented |
| Elevation | Flat | Elevated or depressed |
| Pathologic healing process | None | Hypertrophic scar or keloid |
| Anatomic regions | Flat immobile regions (forearm, thigh) | Mobile curved areas (elbows, knees) |
| Angle of trauma* | Perpendicular angle in hair sparse areas and angular incisions in hair-bearing areas | Angular incisions in hair sparse areas and perpendicular incisions in hair-bearing areas |

**An angled incision causes more injury than a perpendicular injury. An exception to this statement is an angled incision in a less noticeable, hair-bearing area, since there will be less loss of hair in the scar region.*

**Table 2.1** Cosmetically favorable and unfavorable scars

attributed to the underlying soft tissues and rigid bony and cartilaginous structures. Lines of maximum extensibility usually run perpendicular to the RSTLs, meaning that a wound running perpendicular to the lines of maximum extensibility or parallel to the RSTLs will be less obvious and will have a better chance of becoming favorable.

Prior to treatment, the healing potential of patients is important to consider in choosing the ideal treatment for each individual and their scar. Patients with genetic predisposition to keloids and patients with Fitzpatrick's skin types III and above may be poor scar treatment candidates since their outcomes may be worse than their initial scar depending on the treatment chosen (Fig. 2.2). Patients who have used isotretinoin or steroids in the past 6 months may be poor treatment candidates since these medications can impair wound healing, and patients using oral contraceptives or estrogens can have an increased photosensitivity which could cause a postinflammatory mottled appearance and is considered a relative contraindication for chemical peels. Additionally, patients who have problems complying with post-treatment regimens such as minimizing sun exposure, caring for their wounds, or avoiding excessive trauma to wound edges may also be poor treatment candidates for some scar treatments.

Health factors are important to consider for scar treatment candidates. Information should be obtained about the patient's medical history, nutritional status, and ethnicity, which contain factors that can inhibit healing or enhance scarring. Diabetic patients respond more poorly to surgical treatment since they have impaired microvascularization, which hinders wound healing. The nutritional status of the patient is also important since patients with severe vitamin and protein deficiencies will have impaired wound healing (Box 2.1).

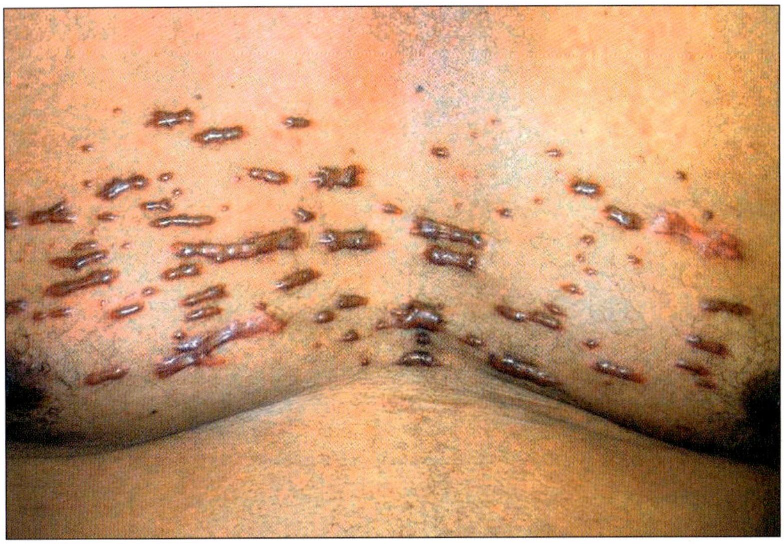

**Fig. 2.2** Keloids on the anterior chest of a dark-skinned individual after inflammatory acne

### Relative Exclusion Criteria for Scar Revision Candidates

Patients who:

- get a lot of sun exposure and do not comply with sunscreen usage or sun exposure restrictions
- have clotting disorders
- have drug allergies
- have used isotretinoin or steroids in the past 6 months
- have nutritional deficiencies
- have uncontrolled diabetes
- cannot properly care for their wounds
- have unresolved psychological distress over the scar
- have unrealistic expectations of the procedure
- are taking postmenopausal estrogens or oral contraceptives
- have a genetic predisposition to keloids
- have Fitzpatrick's skin types of III and above
- have pigmentary disorders
- have Koebnerizing skin conditions
- are unaware of the side effects of the procedures
- have a history of herpes and are unwilling to take antivirals

**Box 2.1** Relative exclusion criteria for scar revision candidates

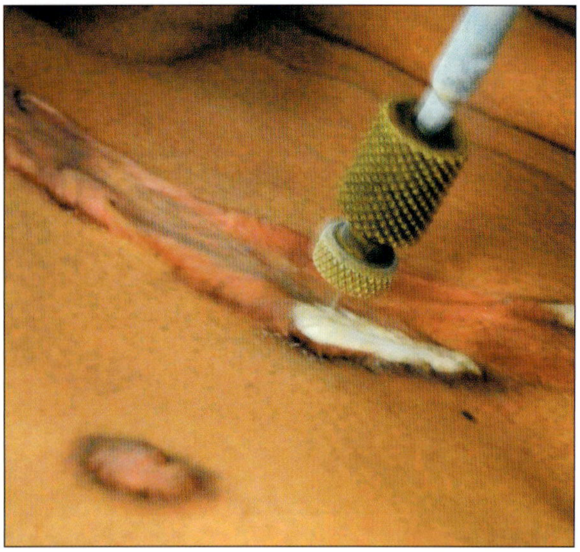

**Fig. 2.3** Liquid nitrogen was applied to the periphery of a large keloid on the anterior chest prior to treatment with intralesional corticosteroid injections

The timing of therapy is important for scar treatment since scars evolve over time. Earlier in the scar remodeling process scars have less tensile strength, and later in the remodeling process the tensile strength increases. For example, at 12–18 months after the injury, scars have the tensile strength of 70–80% of uninjured skin. Therefore, noninvasive procedures such as occlusion therapy or intralesional steroid treatment should be performed within weeks of the scar for better results. However, for invasive procedures such as cryotherapy or surgery, procedures at least 6 months after the formation of the scar have been found to heal better (Fig. 2.3).

## Treatment

### Prevention

Prior to treatment the first rule of thumb with keloids and hypertrophic scars is prevention. Prevention can be both patient and physician oriented. Patients at risk can prevent abnormal scarring from occurring in the first place by avoiding all nonessential cosmetic procedures. Patients prone to abnormal scarring may inform their physician before any surgical intervention so that the physician can take precautionary measures to try and minimize the chances of abnormal scarring. On the other hand, physicians treating areas of trauma with antibiotics and/or anti-inflammatory agents may reduce the chance of abnormal scarring (Table 2.2). Physicians can help prevent abnormal scarring from occurring by minimizing tension and inflammation at all surgical and nonsurgical wound sites, avoiding all incisions on the midchest and joints, and ensuring that when possible, incisions follow skin creases or RSTLs.

| Basic Guidelines for Preventing Abnormal Scarring | |
|---|---|
| **For at-risk patients** | **For physicians** |
| Avoid nonessential surgery and trauma (example: ear piercing, cosmetic surgery) | For all surgical and nonsurgical sites, ensure minimal tension and inflammation |
| Inform physicians of abnormal scarring prior to any procedures | Avoid incisions over the midchest and joints |
| Treat wounds with antibiotics to avoid infections and worsening inflammation | Ensure all wounds follow the skin creases or relaxed skin tension lines |
| Prevent abnormal scarring from occurring by talking to dermatologist about over-the-counter treatments or prescriptions to use for trauma areas | Consider treatments in this chapter to prevent hypertrophic scars and keloids from forming (silicone gel sheeting, nonsilicone occlusion therapy, intralesional corticosteroids) |

**Table 2.2** Basic guidelines for preventing abnormal scarring

## Camouflage and pigmentary therapies

Patients who would like to use noninvasive techniques for treating their scars can use both make-up and pigmentary changing techniques such as pigment lighteners for hyperpigmented scars, and medical tattooing for hypopigmented scars. Opaque make-ups and other cosmetics can conceal erythema, pigment disorders, and scars. Camouflage creams are much heavier and more opaque than regular foundation or powder, and some make-up artists specialize in covering up scars. Accessories and hair can also cover up scars. Chapter 8 focuses on these areas of treatment.

## Occlusion therapy

Occlusion therapy (Fig. 2.4, Box 2.2) includes silicone gels and sheets, nonsilicone occlusive sheets, cordran tape, and Scarguard. Although the mechanism is unknown, silicone treatment has been shown to improve scar contour, color, and texture. It has been proposed that static electricity generated under silicone sheeting could be the reason for its antikeloidal effects. However, in light of the high humidity under occlusive sheeting, it is difficult to generate static electrical charges. Additionally, nonsilicone-based occlusion and hydration have been found to have antikeloidal effects. Occlusion can reduce pro-inflammatory/pro-fibrotic cytokine levels (e.g. interleukin 1 [IL-1]). Increased temperature, even a 1°C change, due to occlusion, can cause significant differences in the collagenase kinetics. Thus, occlusion and hydration can both alter scar remodeling.

Silicone dressings have been widely used since the 1980s. Results from at least eight randomized, controlled trials and a meta-study of 27 trials show that silicone gel sheeting is safe and effective. Studies have shown that silicone gel sheeting with pressure that is worn for up to 12 months for 24 hours a day was found to be effective in treating keloids and/or hypertrophic scars with moderate improvement in

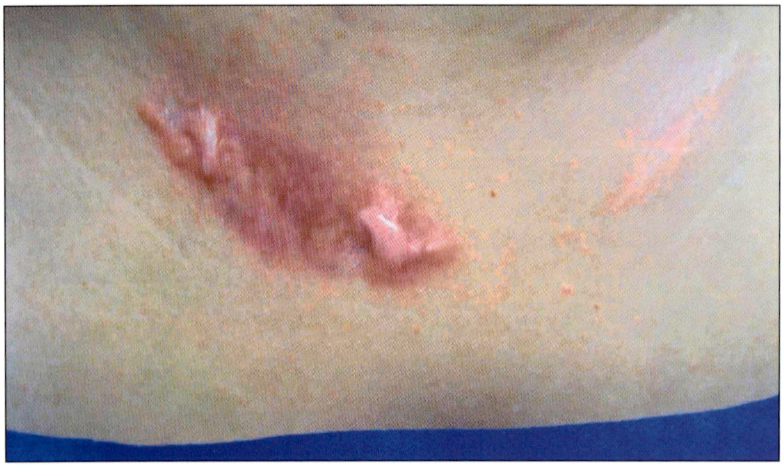

**Fig. 2.4** This keloid on the anterior chest of a light-skinned individual was treated with occlusion therapy to the central portion of the keloid

37.5% and 34% with excellent improvement, while 28% had no or slight improvement.

Studies of nonsilicone occlusive sheets showed mixed results. Nonsilicone occlusive sheets or polyurethane dressing have been shown to soften keloids and cause some regression if worn 20–22 hours a day for at least 8 weeks of therapy. In a study applying semipermeable, semiocclusive, nonsilicone-based dressings to 10 patients for 8 weeks, the results demonstrated: flattening of the keloids (60%), reduced pain (71%), tenderness (78%), pruritus (80%), erythema (87.5%), and satisfaction in 90% of the patients given the treatment. The success rate increases three to four times if pressure is utilized in addition to the occlusion therapy.

Cordran tape has been used for over 30 years for the treatment of hypertrophic scars and keloids. Cordran tape is a clear surgical tape that contains 4 μg of the steroid flurandrenolide and is uniformly distributed evenly on the tape. It has been shown to soften and flatten keloids over time. Its anti-inflammatory properties decrease abnormal scar formation and it is an effective treatment.

Scarguard is a new topical over-the-counter medication containing silicone, hydrocortisone, and vitamin E. An in vitro study showed that Scarguard stimulates the release of inactive collagenase precursors that may inhibit new scars from forming and reduce existing scars. In a pilot study of 12 patients, Scarguard was applied twice daily after the removal of a mole and nothing was applied after the removal of a second mole. After 2 months, nine out of the 12 patients who used Scarguard reported that there was a reduction in the redness and the scar was less noticeable than the scar without treatment.

### *Patients*

Occlusion therapy is appropriate for those patients who would like results without aggressive and painful methods of treatment (Box 2.3,

| Treatment Algorithm for Occlusion Therapy | |
|---|---|
| **Silicone occlusion sheets** | For the use of silicone gel sheets and silicone occlusion sheets, most manufacturers recommend use of the sheets for 12 hours a day up to 3 months. Continued use beyond 3 months may be necessary to maintain its effects. Most of the studies have shown good results with long-term treatment (12 months) with 24 hours a day of usage |
| **Nonsilicone occlusion sheets** | Nonsilicone occlusion therapy has been shown in studies to work with 20–22 hours a day of treatment for at least 2 months |
| **Cordran tape** | Cordran tape (with flurandrenolide incorporated) is used for 12 hours a day with minimal side effects, but can be used up to 24 hours a day for varying amounts of time |
| **Scarguard** | Scarguard is used twice daily for 2–4 months |

**Box 2.2** Treatment algorithm for occlusion therapy

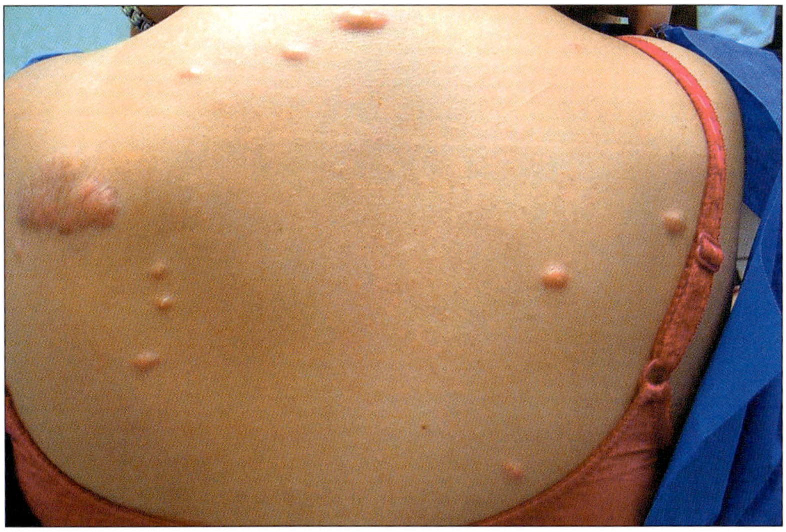

**Fig. 2.5** This young female with keloids from inflammatory acne may respond well to occlusion therapy

> **Indications for Use of Occlusion Therapy**
>
> Occlusion therapy is used in patients who:
>
> - do not want aggressive therapy
> - want to have control over their therapy
> - have or are at risk of getting keloids or hypertrophic scars
> - would like a painless procedure (for example, children)
> - have nonpedunculated keloids
>
> **Equipment:** Desired occlusion product and scissors (to cut the product if needed).

**Box 2.3** Indications for use of occlusion therapy

Fig. 2.5). This therapy is also good for patients who would like control and responsibility with their treatment. For coverage concerns, non-pedunculated keloids work better than pedunculated keloids.

The application of all of these therapies is simple and user friendly. Peel off the back of the sheets and apply them to the affected areas. Some sheets are self-adherent and may be cut to cover the area of concern.

## *Troubleshooting*

The cordran tape has rarely been shown to suppress the hypothalamic–pituitary–adrenal (HPA) axis, or cause manifestations of Cushing's syndrome, hyperglycemia, and glucosuria. With the use of laboratory tests such as urinary cortisol levels and ACTH stimulation tests, a physician can determine if the HPA axis is suppressed. If it is suppressed, the drug should be withdrawn, reduced, or substituted. Also, pediatric populations may absorb steroids more than adults and are more prone to steroid side effects and toxicities. Cordran tape is a pregnancy category C medication.

## *Side effects, complications, and alternative approaches*

Occlusion therapy is painless, however, noncompliance becomes an issue for patients since the treatment is long term. The advantages of occlusion therapy are that: (i) it is easy to use and painless; (ii) usage is only in the area of concern; and (iii) for cordran tape the steroid has an increased penetration in the affected area. The disadvantages of occlusion therapy are that: (i) long-term treatment is often required; (ii) patients need to clean the area and inform their physician if any redness, infection, or itching occurs; (iii) patients need to comply with the medication; and (iv) the results are delayed. Cordran tape has side effects associated with topical steroids. The patient may develop burning, itching, infections, thinning of the skin, blisters, red spots, dry irritated skin, cutaneous atrophy, unusual increased growth of hair, and folliculitis, which is exacerbated by occlusion. Occlusion therapy was used in the central portion of this keloid (Fig. 2.4).

## Compression therapy

Compression therapy is a well-established therapy that has been used since the 1970s. Compression treatments include button compression, pressure earrings, ace bandages, elastic adhesive bandages, compression wraps, lycra bandages, and support bandages. Pressure dressings can be applied directly on the keloid alone or in combination with other treatment modalities such as after the excision of a keloid. The recommended pressure is 24–30 mmHg to exceed the inherent capillary pressure and the suggested treatment time is for 6–12 months. The pressure can be measured with a sphygmomanometer or durometer, however, many of the products are made to reach the specified pressure requirements and the pressure is not usually measured. Often these products can be adjusted for the comfort of the patient.

Mechanistically, pressure results in a reduction of fibroblasts that is most likely caused by tissue hypoxia. Pressure also seems to decrease alpha-macroglobulins that normally inhibit collagenase breakdown of collagen. Another possible mechanism involves decreased scar hydration, resulting in mast cell stabilization, and a reduction in the development of new vasculature and the production of the extracellular matrix.

Efficacy varies depending on the device used. Overall, success rates with pressure therapy have been reported to be in the range of 60–85%. Pressure earrings and button compression demonstrated a 75–100% improvement in 60% of the patients treated. For patients treated with the excision of the keloid and pressure therapy after the excision, a 90–100% 'good' response rate in patients has been reported. The treatment of hypertrophic scars with pressure therapy for several months to 2 years has been shown to resolve hypertrophic scars permanently in a study of 15 patients.

### *Patients*

Compression therapies are used for patients mainly in combination with other treatments such as after a keloid excision, surgical procedures, and burns to prevent keloids or hypertrophic scars from occurring.

### *Equipment*

- Desired pressure product
- Tape or clips, if needed
- Scissors, if needed.

### *Treatment algorithm*

Treatment with pressure therapy is easy. Place the pressure device on top of the affected area to maintain a pressure of 24–30 mmHg for 18–24 hours/day up to 4–6 months or 6–12 months depending on the resource.

### *Troubleshooting*

Nonadherent bandages are less likely to stick to the wound, which would disrupt the healing process.

### *Side effects, complications, and alternative approaches*

There are no known side effects from this medication, however, complications can occur such as ulceration, acne, folliculitis, milia, maceration, infection, and tissue damage to the surrounding skin. Compliance with this treatment modality is an issue for patients since the treatment is long term.

## Corticosteroid injections

Intralesional corticosteroids have been used for scar management since the mid 1960s and are a first-line therapy for keloids. The most common agent is the injection of triamcinolone acetonide in concentrations of 10–40 mg/ml and administered at 4–6-week intervals. The mechanism of action of intralesional corticosteroids is a reduction in the collagen synthesis and glucosaminoglycan synthesis caused by a reduction of the inflammatory mediators and fibroblast proliferation, and increased hypoxia. Intralesional injections of betamethasone sodium phosphate, betamethasone sodium phosphate/betamethasone acetate, triamcinolone diacetate, and triamcinolone hexacetonide have also been used off label for the treatment of keloids, however, triamcinolone acetonide is the treatment of choice.

The efficacy is variable, with a response rate of 50–100% and a reoccurrence rate of 9–50%. Corticosteroids in combination with surgery have had variable reoccurrence rates of 0–100%, with a mean of 50%. As the sole treatment, intralesional corticosteroids appear to be most effective in flattening hypertrophic scars of limited duration. Although keloids injected with corticosteroids may flatten, they often only soften and provide symptomatic relief, a major benefit. The softness or induration of the keloid or hypertrophic scar can be determined by a durometer, which can be cumbersome or suitable for certain body types. Another way of testing induration is with a series of induration disks of known hardness (Fig. 2.6).

### *Patients*

Patients with keloids (Fig 2.7) and hypertrophic scars can be treated with intralesional corticosteroids. Box 2.4 lists the equipment needed to administer this therapy. Nonpedunculated, sessile keloids respond more favorably to intralesional corticosteroids than pedunculated

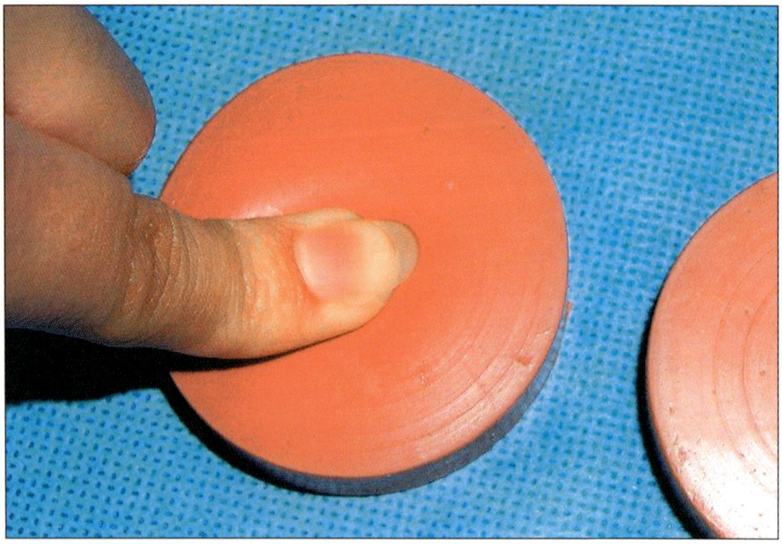

**Fig. 2.6** Induration disks are used to measure the induration of keloids, hypertrophic scars, and other types of scars

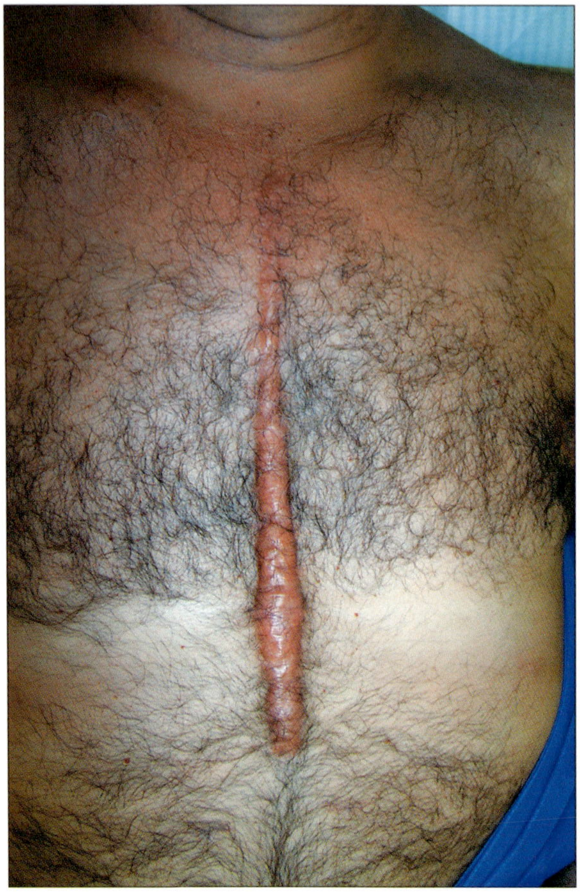

**Fig. 2.7** The keloid found on this light-skinned man formed after coronary bypass surgery. This keloid would be best treated with intralesional steroids. Occlusion therapy would be difficult due to the location of the keloid in a hair-bearing area

### Equipment Needed to Administer Intralesional Corticosteroids

- Needle 25–27 gauge needle
- Corticosteroid of choice with the appropriate concentration for the lesion and at varying amounts (see below)
- 4 × 4 pads
- Anesthetic (optional-lidocaine or cryosurgery)
- Alcohol swabs
- Bandage
- Eye shield (optional)

**Box 2.4** Equipment needed to administer intralesional corticosteroids

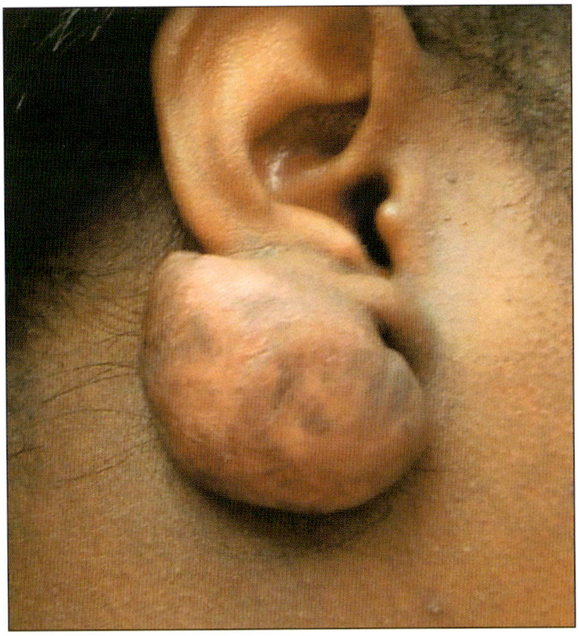

**Fig. 2.8** Pedunculated keloid on a dark-skinned woman years after ear piercing

keloids (Fig. 2.8), which are best treated with surgical excision and adjunctive therapy.

## *Treatment algorithm*

Since the injection can be painful, injecting lidocaine with epinephrine or applying liquid nitrogen can reduce the pain. Keloids can be hard to inject and they may need to be injected several times. If injecting is difficult because of the dense dermal scar, then one option is to use cryotherapy, which causes dermal edema and, thus, facilitates the injection. The intralesional kenalog should be injected into the dermis, where the collagenase is produced, and not into the subcutaneous tissue since this can lead to atrophy. The procedure is as follows:

1. Clean the area with an alcohol pad.
2. Apply anesthesia (optional). Cryosurgery, if used, should be used for 10–15 s to cause cutaneous edema, making it easier to inject a hard keloid (Fig. 2.4).
3. Place fingers on the skin surrounding the keloid and hold the skin taut. Hold the needle with the other hand, making sure that the bevel is facing upward. Some force of the needle may be necessary when injecting a keloid. The needle should be inserted superficially into the keloid and the medication should be injected while removing the syringe. Be careful as you remove the needle since the medication may forcibly spray out as the bevel reaches the surface of the keloid (eye shields can be used for protection). Hypertrophic scars and

softer keloids are not as difficult to inject. Injections are complete when the keloid becomes larger and the color changes to a yellow/white color. This may be difficult to achieve in very hard keloids.

4. After the first injection, check the syringe to see if the needle is clogged.
5. If needed, inject the keloid again until it blanches.

### *Troubleshooting*

The following important points should be borne in mind when troubleshooting:

1. The amount of medication injected into a keloid is a function of the keloid's size, firmness, and location. Although the maximum concentration that should be given is 40 mg/ml, lower concentrations reduce the chance of atrophy and hypopigmentation.
2. It is important to determine if patients are hypertensive or diabetic prior to treating with intralesional steroids and to watch carefully for signs of worsening during the course of their treatment. Other treatment modalities may be used in brittle diabetics and uncontrolled hypertensive patients. Patients with hypertension should check their blood pressure after intralesional steroid injections and be aware that their blood pressure can increase. Diabetics will need to monitor their blood glucose more closely after injections.
3. The concentration used depends on each individual keloid. If the keloid is very hard and firm, a concentration of 40 mg/ml can be used, but it is better to treat it with a lower concentration and evaluate the keloid's response to the treatment to determine what concentration should be used for further treatment.
4. Although the intralesional corticosteroid injection is often painful, similar pain could be felt during anesthetization with lidocaine injections. Local anesthesia is recommended if the keloid is large and needs several injections. Another option is a topical self-warming patch containing lidocaine and tetracaine, which has been shown to decrease the pain of minor dermatologic procedures in a prospectively randomized, double-blinded study (Fig. 2.9).
5. Repeat injections can be performed at 4–6-week intervals. Shorter amounts of time can lead to atrophy since the effects of the prior injection are not complete until 6 weeks after the injection.
6. Inject into the dermis, where collagenase is produced, and not into the subcutaneous tissue since this can lead to underlying fat atrophy.
7. Corticosteroids are given a Pregnancy category C rating (Fig. 2.10).
8. The pediatric dose is not established.

### *Side effects, complications, and alternative approaches*

Side effects of intralesional corticosteroids are: skin atrophy, hyperpigmentation, hypopigmentation, telangiectasia, necrosis, ulceration, and cushingoid features. The risk of these side effects increases if the steroid is injected into the subcutaneous tissue or surrounding dermis.

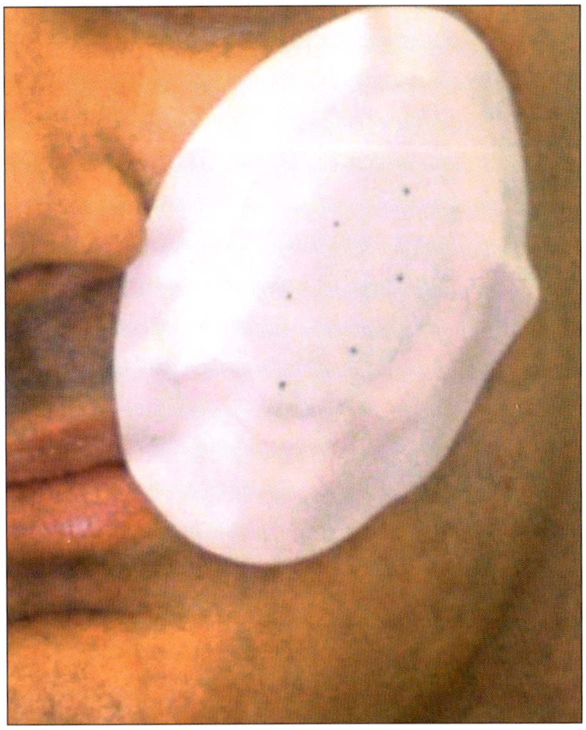

**Fig. 2.9** The Zars patch, a topical self-warming patch containing lidocaine and tetracaine, was used as a local anesthetic on a patient's cheek prior to intralesional corticosteroids

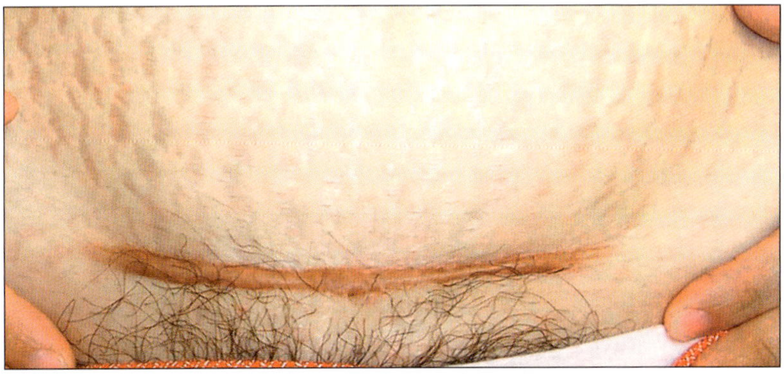

**Fig. 2.10** This keloid on the suprapubic area of a light-skinned female after C-section surgery can be treated with intralesional steroids once the patient has finished breast-feeding her child. Striae distensae can also be seen on the patient's abdomen

Systemic side effects may be seen with large volumes of high-dose corticosteroids. These side effects are: infections, hyperglycemia, edema, osteoporosis, psychosis, growth suppression, osteonecrosis, and peptic ulcer disease; with abrupt discontinuation of the steroids adrenal crises may occur.

## Cryotherapy

Cryotherapy first began in 1899, when Dr White, a dermatologist from the USA, used a cotton applicator in 'liquid air' and utilized it to treat dermatologic conditions. The advent of liquid nitrogen in a spray form over the past century has enhanced the versatility of cryotherapy for dermatologists.

Cryotherapy consists of the freezing of a lesion with the use of liquid nitrogen, causing cell and microvascular damage. Tissue necrosis and sloughing is caused by the anoxia, which leads to tissue flattening. The tissue changes are dependent on the rates of the: temperature fall, rewarming, solute concentration, and length of time the cells are exposed to temperatures below freezing.

The efficacy of cryotherapy varies depending on whether the therapy is used alone or in combination with other treatments. When used alone, 51–74% of patients experienced keloid flattening with two or more sessions of cryotherapy. Additionally, in patients receiving 15–20 s of thawing for eight to 10 visits, each 3 weeks apart, more than half of the patients had complete flattening of their keloids. When used in combination with intralesional corticosteroids, results improved to an 84% response rate. Younger scars and hypertrophic scars responded better to cryotherapy than keloid scars.

### *Patients*

Cryotherapy is not for all patients. Patients with allergies to local anesthetics or anticoagulants, anticipated poor wound healing, and cryoglobulinemia are not good candidates for cryotherapy. Cryotherapy is a blood-free therapy, which is advantageous when treating human immunodeficiency virus (HIV) and hepatitis patients.

### *Equipment*

- Liquid nitrogen
- Cotton swab or a hand-held spray unit
- Pain medication (optional)
- Bandages (optional)

### *Treatment algorithm*

Liquid nitrogen maintained at –195.8°C or –320.4°F, can be applied with a cotton swab, especially for small pedunculated keloids, or with a hand-held spray unit. Unlike the corticosteroid injections, the cryotherapy treatment is dependent mainly on the amount of time of the cryotherapy and less on the clinical appearance of the keloid or hypertrophic scar. Freezing a keloid or a hypertrophic scar can take 10 s to 2 min. No anesthetic preparation is necessary.

### *Troubleshooting*

The following issues should be noted for troubleshooting in using cryotherapy techniques:

1. Pain during and following freezing is more likely when lesions are located on the palms, soles, fingers, toes, scalp, and temple. If pain medication is needed, acetaminophen is used and rarely are other analgesics needed.
2. Bleeding is uncommon but can occur if patients are taking anticoagulants.
3. Syncope infrequently occurs with cryotherapy, but it has been seen when warts are frozen on the fingers. Treating the patient in the prone position is recommended.
4. After cryotherapy, the keloid often may superficially blister or crust over in areas. This is normal and generally not of concern. However, if the area becomes erythematous, warm, tender, and edematous, an infection may be present in a wound created by the cryotherapy, and the patient should be informed to call their dermatologist when this occurs.
5. When using an open container of liquid nitrogen, keep the container on a side table close to the patient and not over the patient in the hands of the an assistant or physician, to avoid spilling the liquid nitrogen.

### *Side effects, complications, and alternative approaches*

The side effects following cryosurgery are pain (this also occurs during the procedure), hyperpigmentation, moderate skin atrophy, edema, vesicles, bullae, weeping, and eschar formation. The common side effect of cryotherapy in keloids is hypopigmentation caused by prolonged freezing times, causing melanocyte destruction. The advantages of cryotherapy are that the infection rates are low and it allows for wounds to heal with little to no scarring. The infection rates are low due to the destruction of the skin flora, maintenance of the basement membrane, and rapid re-epitheliation that occurs with benign and premalignant lesions.

## Soft tissue filler therapy

Soft tissue fillers can augment scars, are generally easy to use, and cause minimal discomfort for the patient. Soft tissue fillers are used for atrophic scars that are pitted or depressed, and due to the ongoing search for the ideal soft tissue filler, many exist with varying usage and side effects.

The two main categories of soft tissue fillers are the biological implants and alloplastic implants. The biological implants that are used for scars include: bovine collagen, autologous collagen, allogenic collagen, autologous fibroblasts, and autologous fat injections. Generally, they have the advantage of having Food and Drug Administration (FDA) approval and the disadvantage of having a lack of permanency and increased hypersensitivity. Alloplastic implants include: silicone, micronized alloderm, polymethylmethacrylate, and polytetrafluoroethylene. They have the advantage of permanency, but they mainly have the disadvantage of not having FDA approval or pending FDA approval, in addition to more side effects.

Soft tissue fillers are used for a variety of indications including wrinkles, scars, atrophic areas, and lip augmentation, and not all of them are utilized for scars. Many soft tissue fillers exist, each with their advantages and disadvantages, emerging almost on a monthly basis. Dermatologists who treat with soft tissue fillers should be aware of all of the different options. The key thing for dermatologists to master is the techniques required for using soft tissue fillers. It is important for dermatologists to feel comfortable using a few of the fillers (Table 2.3) with their different methods required.

### *Patients*

Patients with depressed scars can receive soft tissue fillers. The general exclusion criteria apply (Box 2.1). Patients should also be excluded if the area of interest is infected, but treatment can start once the infection has resolved.

### *Equipment*

- 30 gauge needle (except as noted later)
- Soft tissue filler of choice
- The respective anesthetic

Types of Soft Tissue Fillers Used for the Treatment of Scars

| Collagen | FDA approval | Brand names | Other |
|---|---|---|---|
| **Biologic implants**<br>Bovine collagen | Yes | Zyderm/Zyplast | Bovine (oxen and cow) collagen, bovine collagen derivatives, porcine collagen, hyaluronic acid derivatives |
| Autologous collagen | Yes | Autologen | Processed and harvested from the patient's skin |
| Autologous fibroblasts | Pending | Isolagen | Harvested from human fibroblasts. It was taken off the market in 1999 and is undergoing further tests |
| Autologous fat injection | Yes | Fat | Donor sites include thighs, buttocks, knees, or abdomen |
| **Alloplastic implants**<br>Micronized Alloderm | Yes | Cymetra | An acellular, freeze-dried, dermal graft harvested from screened cadavers |
| Silicone | Yes | Silikon 1000 (off label) | Composed of long polymers of dimethylsiloxanes |
| Polymethylmethacrylate | Pending | Artecoll/Artefill | A suspension of polymethylmethacrylate microspheres in a 3.5% collagen solution with 0.3% lignocaine |
| Polytetraflouroethylene | No | Gore-Tex | A synthetic filler substance (a hollow tube) |

**Table 2.3** Types of soft tissue fillers used for the treatment of scars

### *Treatment algorithm*

A 30-gauge needle is applied at a 45-degree angle while the other hand holds the skin taut. As the needle is withdrawn the soft tissue filler is injected. (Table 2.4) shows the treatment algorithm for use of soft tissue fillers and Table 2.5 the features.

## Chemical peels

Chemical peels (Table 2.6) are an exfoliative process that removes the superficial skin layers and induces epidermal growth and inflammation to establish an organized regrowth of collagen. The three types of chemical peels are: superficial, medium, and deep peels. The superficial peels remove the epidermal layer and have little risk for scarring, but they require weekly to monthly usage for the desired effect. After superficial chemical peels, patients may return to their regular activities and cover the erythematous areas with cosmetics. Medium-depth peels are used for flattening depressed scars, and may be repeated every 3–12 months for desired results. Deep chemical peels can be substituted with laser surgery and dermabrasion for the treatment of scars, with fewer complications and possibly better results.

### *Patients*

Chemical peels are used for patients with depressed and hyperpigmented scars, and other dermatologic conditions such as improving the texture of the skin, reducing hyperpigmentation, wrinkles, acne, rosacea, and melasma.

### *Exclusions/inclusions*

In addition to the general exclusion criteria presented in Box 2.1, the following should be considered:

1. If a patient has received radiation for acne treatment or laser hair removal in the past, adnexal structures must be assessed to ensure adequate epitheliation (vellus hairs or punch biopsy).
2. Patients on medications that make them more photosensitive have relative contraindications for chemical peels. For reference of the most common medications that cause photosensitivity, see Box 2.5.

**Common Medications that Cause Increased Photosensitivity**

- NSAIDs
- Griseofulvin
- Phenothiazines
- Thiazides
- Sulfonamides
- Tetracyclines
- Amiodarone
- Chloroquine
- Methotrexate
- Sulfonylureas
- Flourouuracil
- Vinblastine
- Oral contraceptive pills or estrogen

**Box 2.5** Common medications that cause increased photosensitivity

## Superficial peels

Superficial peels come in a variety of forms as seen in Table 2.6. Trichloroacetic acid (TCA) 10–35% concentration is used for superficial peels and comes in paste or liquid forms. Modified Unna's resorcinol paste 10–30% is also used for superficial peels.

Jessner's solution is a mixture of resorcinol 14%, salicylic acid 14%, and lactic acid 14% in ethanol. It is used with either light or heavy applications and may be repeated every 3–4 minutes for desired results. Salicylic acid is used in a 50% solution for superficial peels and

| Treatment Algorithms of Soft Tissue Fillers | | | | | | |
|---|---|---|---|---|---|---|
| **Category** | **Skin testing** | **Anesthesia** | **Injection** | **Overcorrection** | **Lasts** | **Indication** |
| Bovine: Zyderm Zyplast | Yes, 2 and 6 weeks prior to injections | Contains lidocaine topical anesthetic or nerve blocks may be added | Zyderm: injected into the superficial papillary dermis Zyplast: injected into the midreticular deep reticular dermis | Zyplast does not require overcorrection but Zyderm I and Zyderm II require 200% and 150% overcorrection respectively | 3–6 months | Zyderm: I and II scars Zyplast: deep scars |
| Autologous: Autologen | No | Need nerve blocks, topical or local anesthesia | Injections last 3–6 months | Yes, by 20–30% | >18 months | Atrophic scars |
| Allogenic: Dermalogen | No | Need nerve blocks, topical or local anesthesia | Around three injections are required over several weeks | Yes, by 20–30% | 4–6 months | Atrophic scars |
| Autologous Fibroblasts: Isolagen | Yes, 2 weeks prior | Unknown (off the market) | Injections into the mid-upper dermis every 2 weeks for a total of 3 injections | Yes, by 300% | Unknown | Scars |
| Autologous fat injection | No | Tumescent anesthesia is given | *16–18 gauge needle | Yes, 50–85% | >1 year | Depressed atrophic areas, scars |
| Micronized Alloderm: Cymetra | Yes | It is mixed with lidocaine | *26 gauge needle, injected into subdermis | Yes, 30% | 4–6 months | Scars, atrophic areas, burns |
| Silicone | No | Need topical anesthetic | Injected in microdroplets of 0.01 ml into subdermis | No, under-correction is needed. | Permanent | Scars |
| Polymethyl-methacrylate: Artecoll/Artefill | Yes, 4 and 2 weeks prior | Added to lidocaine | *27 gauge needle, injected into subdermis | Yes, slight overcorrection | 1 year | Atrophic scars |
| Polytetra-fluoroethylene: Gore-Tex | No | Need local anesthesia | Threaded through a guiding needle into deep dermis | No | Permanent | Deep defects |

**All soft tissue fillers use a 30 gauge needle except for the starred ones with their respective gauge needle required specified.*

**Table 2.4** Treatment algorithms of soft tissue fillers

| Features of Soft Tissue Fillers | | | | |
|---|---|---|---|---|
| **Category** | **Advantages** | **Disadvantages** | **Complications** | **Troubleshooting** |
| Bovine: Zyderm Zyplast | Long track record and safety profile, easy use, readily available, performed in an office, reasonable cost, minimal pain | Impermanence, must be refrigerated, hypersensitivity reactions, requires two skin tests. If Zyderm is injected too deep then the injection is lost, and if it is injected too superficially then white material will show | Bruising, reactivation of herpes virus, bacterial infections, local necrosis, intermittent swelling, and cystic reactions | 1. Perform a stretch test* 2. Avoid ASA, NSAIDs, vitamin E, green tea, and other anticoagulants 10 days prior to treatment 3. If bruising occurs, add topical vitamin K |
| Autologous: Autologen | No skin testing is necessary, longlasting effects, collagen injected is from patient's own skin, no risk of disease transmission | Requires additional surgery for skin sample needed to make the Autologen Material must be sent away for processing. Either a dermatologic surgeon or plastic surgeon is needed. Expensive, pain with injection, lack of permanency, extra time for harvesting | Bruising, swelling, tenderness, infection | Avoid ASA, NSAIDs, vitamin E, green tea, and other anticoagulants 10 days prior to treatment |
| Autologous fibroblasts: Isolagen | There are no reported allergic reactions | A postauricular skin biopsy is necessary. Injection is required within 48 hours of the receipt of the material. Long processing time, skin testing, high cost, pain with injection, delayed improvement | Bruising, swelling, tenderness, infection | Avoid ASA, NSAIDs, vitamin E, green tea, and other anticoagulants 10 days prior to treatment |
| Autologous fat injection | No skin testing is required, unlimited supply, no cost for the product | A larger needle is needed because of the higher viscosity of the fluid, which causes more pain and a visible puncture hole that may last for days<br>Donor site morbidity, calcification of the injected fat, unpredictable resorption | Increased swelling, bruising, and tenderness because a larger needle is needed<br>Undercorrection and overcorrection, irregularities, infection, necrosis | Fat implantations are more successful in the face, where there is more vasculature |
| Micronized Alloderm: Cymetra | No skin testing is required | Longevity is unknown, long preparation time, harder technique to implant the filler | Bruising, swelling, tenderness, infection | Avoid ASA, NSAIDs, vitamin E, green tea, and other anticoagulants 10 days prior to treatment |
| Silicone | Easy to use, permanent, inexpensive | It has been associated with multiple side effects and bad outcomes, delayed hypersensitivity, painful injections | Hypersensitivity, granuloma formation, migration of the material, swelling, induration, discoloration, ulceration, bumpiness, death | Nonphysicians have used this in the past with tainted silicone injections and have caused death of one patient |

**Table 2.5** Features of soft tissue fillers

| Features of Soft Tissue Fillers (*Cont'd*) | | | | |
|---|---|---|---|---|
| **Category** | **Advantages** | **Disadvantages** | **Complications** | **Troubleshooting** |
| Polymethyl-methacrylate: Artecoll/Artefill | Longer lasting correction | Higher price because of the processing, greater trauma with a larger needle, two skin tests are recommended | Edema, bruising, tenderness, granuloma formation and cystic nodules have been observed. Swelling, pain, persistent erythema, visible or palpable granules, purities, hypertrophic scarring at injection sites | 1. It is easy to inject too much, therefore be careful when injecting. 2. Gently massage the area after injection. 3. Tape should be placed over the treated area for 2 days until the microspheres are fixed in place by fibrous tissue |
| Polytetra-flouroethylene: Gore-Tex | Effects are immediate and permanent, implant is removable, no skin tests are needed | Additional training is required, a course of antibiotics is recommended | Extrusion or open-air exposure, granulomas, post-inflammatory skin infections | 1. If an infection occurs, the Gore-Tex needs to be removed 2. NSAIDs, ASA, vitamin E and green tea should be avoided 10 days prior to implantation to decrease the chances of bruising |

**Stretch test: Not all depressed scars respond to bovine injections, but a stretch test can help determine if the scar will respond. If the skin surrounding the scar is stretched and the scar flattens, then the scar can be corrected with bovine injections.*

**Table 2.5** (*Cont'd*) Features of soft tissue fillers

may be used under an occlusive dressing that can be removed after 48 h. Salicylic acid peels may be repeated every 2–4 weeks. Alpha-hydroxy acids (AHAs) such as glycolic acids and lactic acids are applied rapidly, in a 20-second period with a cotton applicator. Results become unpredictable with excessive rubbing, so careful application must be performed. Beta-hydroxy acids (BHAs), such as salicylic acid, are used at 20–30% for chemical peels. Both AHAs and BHAs are used for hyperpigmented scars, not depressed scars.

## Medium-depth peels

Medium-depth peels use the same solutions as in the superficial peels, but they are used at greater concentrations or in combination with other chemicals. TCA is used for medium-depth peels at a 35–40% concentration. Combination treatments include solid carbon dioxide ($CO_2$) or dry ice, Jessner's solution or glycolic acid prior to 35% TCA. This treatment can be used for both medium-depth and deep chemical peels. When dry ice or solid $CO_2$ is used for medium-depth peels,

| Types of Chemical Peels | |
|---|---|
| **Superficial** | **Medium** |
| TCA 10–35% concentration | TCA 35–40% concentration |
| Modified Unna's Resorcinol Paste 10–30% | Combination treatment (see page 37) |
| Jessner's Solution | |
| Salicylic acid 50% solution | |
| AHAs and BHAs | |

**Table 2.6** Types of chemical peels

it should be wrapped in a hand towel and dipped in a 3:1 acetone and alcohol solution and applied to the skin. The combination treatments avoid the increased scarring and hypopigmentation that is seen with higher concentrations of TCA. Jessner's solution can be applied numerous times to achieve more epidermal interruption, and glycolic acid (usually 70%) can be left on the skin longer to achieve more epidermolysis. After the superficial agent, the TCA is applied until a frosting appears, a grayish-white appearance of the skin.

### *Equipment*

- Anesthesia (including meperidine (demerol), midazolam (versed), or diazepam (valium) for the patient, if needed)
- Cotton or gauze
- Acid of choice for exfoliation
- Cooling devices – handheld fan, ice, dry ice
- Moisturizer of choice
- Water in a bowl and sodium bicarbonate for neutralization

Box 2.6 outlines the procedure for examination at follow-up visits and Box 2.7 details the treatment algorithm for administering chemical peels.

### *Troubleshooting*

1. Phenol can cause renal and cardiac abnormalities. Be aware that hydration is needed to prevent these side effects. Hydration is not required for the application of phenol on one cosmetic area or less. For phenol peels on more than one cosmetic subunit, 8–16 oz of water may be given prior to the procedure. Additionally, Ringer's lactate may be given prior to, during, and after the phenol peel.
2. Do not use emulsifiers or additives to TCA that could increase its penetration to the lower dermis.
3. Patients should be shown pictures of what they will look like after the peel to know what to expect, especially during the healing phase.

### *Side effects, complications, and alternative approaches*

1. The overall side effects of all superficial peels are: erythema, itching, peeling, increased skin sensitivity, and epidermolysis. Post-inflammatory hyperpigmentation is rare in superficial peels.
2. AHAs and BHAs. The advantages of AHAs are that the results are slow and complications are rare, and the disadvantages are that results are slow and often minimal. The advantages of BHAs are that: there is minimal edema and erythema, there is no need to neutralize BHAs like the AHAs, and a frost is visible once the peel is complete, making it easy to identify areas that were not treated. BHAs can be used in large areas of the body for hyperpigmented scars since it does not require neutralization, however, large areas of the body should not be treated at once since toxic levels of salicylic

| Follow-up Visits Should Consist of: | |
|---|---|
| Day 1 | Make sure the postoperative regimen is clear and that everything is going smoothly |
| Day 3 | Look for signs of infection |
| Day 7 | Check for completion of the peel. The lotion regimen may need to be changed to something lighter at this time |
| Week 3 | Make sure there is no rebound hyperpigmentation. Bleaching agents can be used to hasten any hyperpigmentation. Check if any persistent erythema exists. If there is persistent erythema these areas need to be watched closely to make sure no scars form. These areas may need to be treated with topical steroids. |
| Month 3 | Check the healing process (physically and histologically). If needed, plan for ancillary treatments such as the use of monthly glycolic acid peels to help refine the results of the dermal peel |

**Box 2.6** Follow-up visits

**Treatment Algorithm for Chemical Peels**

**Before the chemical peel**

- First figure out where the line of demarcation should lie, at the mandible for a facial peel or the chest for a facial and neck peel. The line of demarcation will be visible especially in patients with freckles and dark colored skin
- Daily sunscreen use and nightly tretinoin should be used to reduce solar pigmentation and promote faster healing after the peel. Tretinoin does not enhance the efficacy of the peel
- Some dermatologists use hydroquinone gel 4% or kojic acid twice daily for one month before the peel to both test the patients' reactivity to the product and begin bleaching of the epidermal pigment. It may cause ochronosis in patients with Fitzpatrick types V and VI skin

**Steps of the chemical peel**

- Degrease the face by removing cutaneous lipids with alcohol or acetone-soaked sponges
- Divide the face into six regions: forehead, perioral, right and left cheeks, nose, and periorbital region
- When using Jessner's solution, apply a thin layer of petroleum jelly or Auquaphor to the areas that are not intended to get treated
- Apply the peel solution to each area in the following order: forehead, perioral, right and left cheeks, nose, and periorbital region. Each section should be treated with 10–15 minutes between sections, thus taking 60–90 minutes for the entire face. Use cotton swabs to apply the acid solution when less penetration and minimal mechanical effect is desired. Use soaked gauze pads when deeper penetration is needed. Applying more coats adds to the depth of the penetration. This may be needed in areas of thicker skin, but care is needed because unintended deeper penetration can result in scars
- Neutralize the area with 10% sodium bicarbonate when the desired endpoint has been reached. The desired endpoint for the patient may be when a frost occurs on the skin, or a whitish/gray color appears. Some solutions do not need neutralization (see later)
- If tape is indicated, tape can be placed after the peel and removed in 48 hours

**After the chemical peel**

- Wet to dry dressings are used three to five times a day using water, half strength boric acid, or dilute antiseptic providence-iodine skin cleanser. An occlusive moisturizer like petroleum can also be used
- Sunscreen should be used for at least one month after the peel to protect the skin

**Box 2.7** Treatment algorithm for chemical peels

acid can accumulate and patients can experience nausea, disorientation, and tinnitus. BHAs are contraindicated in patients who are allergic to aspirin, pregnant, or breast-feeding. The disadvantage of both AHAs and BHAs is that patients are susceptible to increased photosensitivity. Sunscreen should always be used with these treatments. Also, extra care must be taken when using the acid solutions around the eyes since they can cause significant damage to the cornea.

3. The advantages of Jessner's solution are: that a single solution is needed, no neutralizing agents are required, and it amplifies the effects of 5-fluorouracil (5-FU). The disadvantages associated with Jessner's peels are that postinflammatory hyperpigmentation may occur in darker skinned patients (Fitzpatrick skin type IV and greater) and the patient may experience flaking for approximately 7 days.
4. The healing time for peels is 7 days for patients with the TCA peels and 7–10 days for patients treated with a combination of TCA and Jessner's peel or glycolic acid peels. TCA peel patients will look terrible after the peel. On days 1 and 2 the skin appears pink, on days 3 and 4 the skin darkens, and on days 5–10 the skin peels off. Erythema may last until day 14. Streaking can also appear around

the margins of the peeled areas, therefore, careful application of the TCA is necessary.

5. For better results, chemical peels can be used with $CO_2$ laser resurfacing and dermabrasion.

See Box 2.8 for adverse reactions to use of chemical peels.

## New Treatments

### Verapamil

Verapamil is a calcium channel blocker and blocks the synthesis/secretion of extracellular matrix molecules (collagen, glycosaminoglycans, fibronectin, and fibrinase). A study was conducted of 22 patients with keloids who were treated with surgical excision and five treatments of verapamil 2.5 mg/ml (doses varied from 0.5–5 ml depending on the size of the keloid) over a 2-month period. These patients were evaluated at a 2-year follow up point. Two patients had keloids that decreased in size from the original lesion, two patients had hypertrophic scars, four patients had pruritis, and one patient had a keloid on the donor site.

### Intralesional bleomycin

Injections of bleomycin cause necrosis of keratinocytes with a mixed inflammatory infiltrate. In two studies, bleomycin was used to treat keloids and hypertrophic scars. In one study, bleomycin was given at a concentration of 1.5 IU/ml to 13 patients using the multiple-puncture method; bleomycin was dripped onto the lesion and then multiple punctures were made on the lesions by means of a syringe. Seven patients had complete flattening of their lesions, five had highly significant flattening, and one patient had significant flattening. In another study of 31 keloids, patients were treated with 3–5 infiltrates of bleomycin within a 1-month period. Total regression occurred in 84% of the keloids tested and reduction occurred in the keloid volume and functional impairment.

### Intralesional 5-fluorouracil (5-FU)

5-FU, a pyrimidine analog, inhibits fibroblastic proliferation in tissue culture and is believed to reduce postoperative scarring by decreasing fibroblast proliferation. 5-FU has also been shown to be safe and effective in the treatment and prevention of hypertrophic scars with some responsiveness in small keloids.

Three studies have shown the effectiveness of 5-FU. In one prospective, randomized, uncontrolled trial, 28 patients were treated with weekly injections of 0.5–2.0 ml at a 50 mg/ml concentration of 5-FU for 12 weeks, and at the 24-week follow up, 70% of the patients had a result of more than a 50% improvement in keloid size. In the other retrospective study of 1000 patients treated with hypertrophic scars and keloids over a 9-year period, the most effective regimen was found to be 0.1 ml of triamcinolone acetonide (10 mg/ml) and 0.9 ml of

## Adverse Reactions Associated with the Chemical Peel

**Infections (viral, *Candida*, bacterial)**

- Prophylactic treatment is needed for herpes (acyclovir 400 mg p.o. b.i.d.), even in patients without a history of recurrent herpes simplex
- Hyperpigmentation
- Hypopigmentation is seen with the use of phenol, and is usually proportional to the amount of phenol used
- Milia, acne, cyst formation
- Occlusive ointments and acne prone skin contributes to these problems. Treatment with acne preparations, oral antibiotics, and intralesional steroids may be helpful

**Unaffected areas (perioral region)**

Since lip and mouth protection is important, gauze can be placed between the lips and petroleum jelly can be placed on and around the lips to avoid any excess acid from damaging this area. When the perioral region is not treated with the peel then it can be blended in with the rest of the face by using additional treatments with lasers, dermabrasion, or deep phenol peels

- Infections (viral, *Candida*, bacterial)
- Prophylactic treatment is needed for herpes (acyclovir 400 mg p.o. b.i.d.) even in patients without a history of recurrent herpes simplex

**Hyperpigmentation**

- Early use of hydroquinones and low potency steroids usually help the problem. It usually occurs in dark skin patients that receive chemical peels and is caused by sunlight, estrogen, photosensitizing drugs, and pregnancy

**Hypopigmentation**

- Hypopigmentation is seen with the use of phenol, and it is usually proportional to the amount of phenol used

**Milia, acne, cyst formation**

- Occlusive ointments and acne prone skin contributes to these problems. Treatment with acne preparations, oral antibiotics, and intralesional steroids may be helpful

**Erythema**

- Persistent erythema may be the early signs of a scar. Early use of medium to high potency steroids is important prior to the scar development. Patients should avoid isotretinoin and alcoholic beverages after the chemical peels since increased erythema can occur. Patients with rosacea and contact dermatitis may also have increased redness after chemical peels

**Scars**

- If a scar develops, then pulse dye laser therapy can be used, but delaying any subsequent surgery for 1 year after the procedure has been recommended

**Pain**

- For pain relief use: oral diazepam, stationary or handheld fans, EMLA and ELAMAX, ice and water packs (immediately after the peel), and/or an ointment to relieve pain both during and after the procedure. Anesthetics and nerve blocks can be used in medium and deep chemical peels

**Crusting**

- To minimize crusting after a peel, use wet to dry soaks of tap water or skin cleansers twice daily
- Unaffected areas (perioral region): Since lip and mouth protection is important, gauze can be placed between the lips and petroleum jelly can be placed on and around the lips to avoid any excess acid from damaging this area. When the perioral region is not treated with the peel then it can be blended in with the rest of the face by using additional treatments with lasers, dermabrasion, or deep phenol peels

**Contact dermatitis**

- Irritant contact dermatitis has been reported in the following peeling agents: resorcinol, salicylic acid, kojic acid, lactic acid, and hydroquinone

**Box 2.8** Adverse reactions associated with the chemical peel

5-FU (50 mg/ml) injections up to three times a week. A total of 20 patients with keloids were treated with 5-FU (50 mg/ml) once weekly with an average of seven treatments; 85% of these patients had greater than a 50% improvement of their keloids, however 47% of the patients had reoccurrence within 1 year. The main adverse events included pain, hyperpigmentation, and tissue sloughing.

## Topical retinoic acid

Retinoic acid decreases normal tonofilament and keratohyalin synthesis, increases production of mucoid substances and epidermal cell growth rate, and inhibits DNA synthesis in vitro. In a clinical trial involving 21 patients with 28 keloids and hypertrophic scars, retinoic acid was applied for at least 3 months twice daily and showed favorable results in 77–79% of the lesions tested, including a decrease in the size and symptoms of the scar.

## Imiquimod

Imiquimod 5% cream has been approved by the FDA for the treatment of external genital and perianal warts, actinic keratosis, and superficial basal cell carcinoma. Imiquimod induces TNF-alpha, IFN-alpha and gamma, and IL-1, 6, 8, and 12, and alters the expression of markers for apoptosis. In one study, 13 keloids were treated with excision and imiquimod was applied every night for 8 weeks. Ten patients with 11 keloids completed the 6-month study, and no recurrences occurred after 6 months. Mild irritation was experienced with application of the imiquimod, and some patients needed a cessation period from the medication. Hyperpigmentation was experienced by more than half of the patients in the study.

## Interferon therapy

Interferon alpha (INF-$\alpha$), -$\beta$, and -$\gamma$ have been used in in vitro studies to reduce the synthesis of collagen types I, III, and possibly VI via a reduction in a cellular ribonucleic acid. Intralesional IFN-$\alpha$2b has been found to reduce the size of nonsurgically excised keloids. In a clinical trial, there was a statistically significant decrease in the recurrence of 124 excised keloids when administering post-excision interferon $\alpha$-2b (18.7% recurrence) vs. excision alone (51.1%), vs. treatment with postoperative intralesional triamcinolone (58.4%). Acetaminophen is recommended in large excision sites to help negate the flu-like symptoms caused by interferon.

## Tacrolimus

Tacrolimus is an immunomodulator that inhibits TNF-$\alpha$. Gli-1, an oncogene, has been found to be overexpressed in fibroblasts of keloids. Rapamycin, a close analogue of tacrolimus was used in an in vitro study and was found to inhibit the gli-1 oncogene, thus, giving a rationale to initiate clinical trials of topical tacrolimus and rapamycin. In an open-label pilot study, 11 patients used tacrolimus 0.1% ointment on their keloids twice daily for 12 weeks. Although the results were not statistically significant, the study showed a decrease in the induration, tenderness, erythema, and pruritus in most of the patients.

## Botulinum toxin

Botulinum toxin A is a potent drug that produces temporary muscular paralysis when injected locally, and in a randomized, double-blind, placebo-controlled primate study the wounds that were immobilized with the botulinum toxin were significantly better than the controlled wounds. In two case studies involving patients who used botulinum toxin on postoperative wounds, the wounds healed more favorably and no side effects were experienced.

## Further Reading


Baumann L 2002 Chemical peels. In: Weisberg E (ed) Cosmetic Dermatology: Principles and Practice. McGraw Hill, New York, pp 173–186

Baumann L 2002 Soft tissue fillers. In: Weisberg E (ed) Cosmetic Dermatology: Principles and Practice. McGraw Hill, New York, pp 155–172

Beckenstein MS, Kuniaki T, Matarasso A 2004 The effect of Scarguard on collagenase levels using a full-thickness epidermal model. Aesthetic Surgery Journal 24:1–5

Berman B, Flores F 1999 Comparison of a silicone gel-filled cushion and silicon gel sheeting for the treatment of hypertrophic or keloid scars. Dermatologic Surgery 25:484–486

Berman B, Flores J, Pariser D, Pariser R, De Araujo T, Ramirez CC 2005 Self-warming lidocaine/tetracaine patch effectively and safely induces local anesthesia during minor dermatologic procedures. Dermatologic Surgery 31:135–138

Berman B, Kapoor S 2002 Keloids and hypertrophic scars. eMedicine July 12, www.emedicine.com/derm/topic205.htm

Berman B, Poochareon V, Villa AM. An open-label, pilot study to evaluate safety and tolerability of keloid treatment with tacrolimus ointment 0.1%. (in press)

Berman B, Romagosa R, Zell D 2004 Keloid scarring, treatment of skin disease. In: Lebwohl M, Heyman W, Berth-Jones J, Coulson I Comprehensive Therapeutic Strategies. 2nd edn. (in press)

Brody HJ 1999 Skin resurfacing: chemical peels. In: Freedberg IM, Eisen AZ, Wolff K et al (eds) Fitzpatrick's Dermatology in General Medicine. 5th edn. McGraw Hill, New York, 1999, 2937–2946

Busso M 2004 New Injectable Tissue Fillers. H & H Dermatological Society South Beach Conference 2004 lecture notes

Cheng JT, Perkins SW, Hamilton MM 2002 Collagen and injectable fillers. Otolaryngology Clinics of North America 35:73–85, vi

Coleman WP III 2001 Dermal peels. Dermatology Clinics 19(3):405–411

Eisen D 2004 A pilot study to evaluate the efficacy of Scarguard in the prevention of scars. Internet Journal of Dermatology 5(2):

Flores J, Berman B, Burdick A, Jonusas AM 1998 The effectiveness of a new method for assessing induration. Journal of the American Academy of Dermatology 39(6):1021–1022

Goodman GJ 2000 Postacne scarring: a review of its pathophysiology and treatment. Dermatologic Surgery 26:857–871

Graham GF 1999 Cryosurgery. In: Freedberg IM, Eisen AZ, Wolff K, et al (eds) Fitzpatrick's Dermatology in General Medicine. 5th edn. McGraw Hill, New York, pp 2980–2987

Kontochristopoulos G, Stefanaki C, Panagiotopoulos A, et al 2005 Intralesional 5-fluorouracil in the treatment of keloids: An open clinical and histopathologic study. Journal of the American Academy of Dermatology 52(3 Part 1):474–479

Kotler HS 2002 Scar revision. eMedicine July 16

Lyle WG 2001 Silicone gel sheeting. Plastic Surgery Educational Foundation DATA Committee. Plastic and Reconstructive Surgery 107:272–275

Moran ML 2001 Management of facial cutaneous defects. Part II. Otolaryngologic Clinics of North America 34:1–10

Mustoe TA, Cooter RD, Gold MH, et al 2002 International clinical recommendations on scar management. International Advisory Panel on Scar Management. Plastic and Reconstructive Surgery 110(2):560–571

Niessen FB, Spauwen PH, Schalkwijk J, Kon M 1999 On the nature of hypertrophic scars and keloids: a review. Plastic and Reconstructive Surgery 104:1435–1458

Porter JP 2002 Treatment of the keloid: what is new? Otolaryngology Clinics of North America 35:207–220, viii

Young AM, Tan PJ, Berman B, Villa AM, Poochareon V 2002 Topical application of a semipermeable, semiocclusive, non-silicone-based dressing for keloid treatment. Cosmetic Dermatology 15:33–34

# 3 Surgical Approaches to Patients with Scarring

*Joanna Mimi Choi, Thomas E. Rohrer, Michael S. Kaminer, R. Sonia Batra*

## Introduction

'Doc, I hate this scar. Can you do anything about it?' is a request often made by people with conspicuous scars. A successful scar revision can markedly improve quality of life for these patients. While surface defects cannot be completely erased, dermatologists can employ a wide variety of surgical approaches to help replace existing scars with more esthetically pleasing ones.

Scar formation is a normal and necessary process for the healing of tissue after insult. However, abnormal healing or disturbed collagen production can result in an inadequate restoration of the cutaneous surface and permanent textural irregularities. A scar generally achieves a steady state after 1 year and will ultimately reach only 80% of the tensile strength of normal skin.

Clinically, a cosmetically acceptable scar is level with the surrounding skin, soft, a good color match, and narrow. Favorable lines of closure are often within or parallel to relaxed skin tension lines (RSTLs), lines due to the dynamic action of the underlying musculature (Fig. 3.1). Preoperative planning and prevention are critical to achieving scar cosmesis. Moreover, a clear understanding of the types of abnormal scars a dermatologist may face and the arsenal of surgical approaches to revise them are of immense benefit in the battle against 'ugly' scars.

This chapter will focus on surgical methods for scar revision. For information on the use of lasers and other adjunctive therapies in scar revision, please refer to the appropriate sections of this volume.

## Types of Clinical Scars

From an etiologic perspective, there are four main categories of scars that may require revision: (i) poorly designed; (ii) arising from trauma; (iii) poorly healed; and (iv) disease related (Table 3.1). The resulting scar abnormality guides the choice of revision technique (Table 3.2).

Poorly designed scars do not lie within RSTLs or along cosmetic unit junctions and/or do not respect facial landmarks or free tissue margins such as the lip or eyelid. Consequently, they are not well camouflaged and are especially apparent to the observer. The appearance of these scars varies broadly, presenting as elevated, depressed, widened,

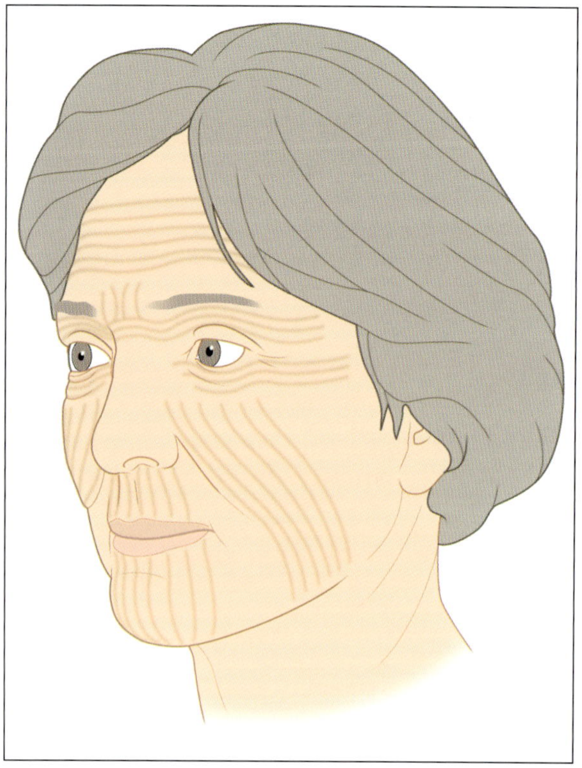

**Fig. 3.1** RSTLs due to dynamic action of the underlying facial musculature. Lines are often perpendicular to muscle fibers. Incisions should be parallel or within RSTLs for optimal scar cosmesis

| Etiologic Categories for Abnormal Scars | |
|---|---|
| **Category** | **Examples of causes** |
| Poorly designed | Not parallel or within RSTLs<br>Lack of respect for facial landmarks<br>Long linear design<br>Depressed scars from lack of evertional closure |
| Traumatic or irregular wound creation | Burn<br>Debris |
| Prior poor healing | Infection<br>Excess tension<br>Necrosis or slough |
| Disease related | Acne<br>Varicella<br>Keloid |

**Table 3.1** Etiologic categories for abnormal scars

| Scar Abnormalities and Treatment Approaches | | |
|---|---|---|
| **Scar Abnormality** | **Causes** | **Treatment methods** |
| *Elevated* | Wound closure under tension<br>Inadequate apposition of wound edges<br>Full-thickness grafts (commonly oversized) | Intralesional corticosteroids<br>Shave excision<br>Fusiform excision<br>Dermabrasion<br>Laser resurfacing |
| *Hypertrophic scars/keloids* | Genetic predisposition<br>Area of motion or tension<br>Nidus of prolonged inflammation (e.g. infection or foreign body reaction) | Intralesional corticosteroids<br>Shave excision<br>Fusiform excision<br>Radiation<br>Cryosurgery<br>Lasers<br>Compression therapy |
| *Depressed scar* | Deep shave biopsy<br>Electrodessication/curettage<br>Deficient wound eversion<br>Wound healing complicated by hematoma or infection | Fusiform excision and suture w/ buried vertical mattress intradermal sutures<br>Fillers<br>Subcision/subdermal undermining |
| *Widened scars* | Wounds closed under tension | Excision and suture w/ buried vertical mattress intradermal sutures |
| *Long linear scar* | Preoperative poor planning | W-plasty<br>Geometric broken line closure<br>Dermabrasion |
| *Pitted/ice pick* | Prior acne<br>Trauma | Punch excision<br>Punch grafting<br>Dermal pocket grafting<br>Dermabrasion |
| *Contracted/webbed* | Traverse concavities | Z-plasties |

**Table 3.2** Scar abnormalities and treatment approaches

contracted, webbed, or long and linear. A schematic diagram of different scar types is presented in Figure 3.2. Traumatic scars often do not follow good scar design, as they arise from accidental events such as burns or lacerations, and do not have the benefit of careful preoperative planning. Furthermore, by contraction, burns may increase skin tension and result in a thin atrophic dermis. Fortunately, a simple fusiform excision or scar irregularization can help to better camouflage these scars within RSTLs.

Poor healing from infection, excess wound tension, presence of a foreign body, or necrosis with slough can also create disfiguring scars, especially keloidal or hypertrophic scars. A keloid invades beyond the boundaries of the original wound and is often painful and pruritic. This scar type develops a median of 30.4 months after injury and can often

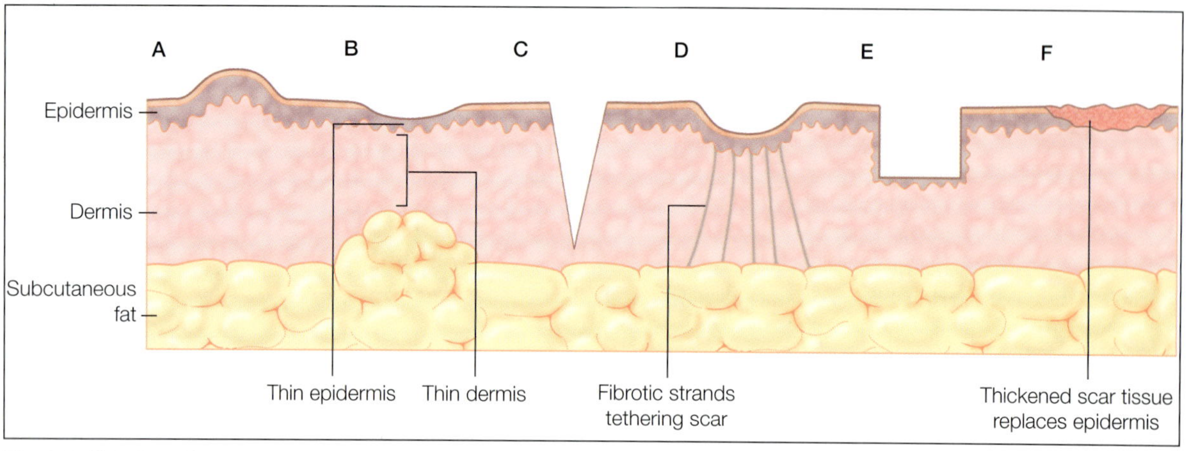


**Fig. 3.2** Sideview of scar subtypes. (**A**) Elevated scar. (**B**) Atrophic scar with thinning of epidermis and dermis. (**C**) Ice pick or pitted scar. (**D**) Rolling scar. Note fibrous tethers. (**E**) Boxcar scar. (**F**) Contracted or webbed scar. Thickened scar tissue replaces normal epidermis

recur, especially in high-risk sites such as the shoulders, chest, earlobes, upper arms, and cheeks. While the hypertrophic scar also has a raised appearance, its size is limited to the boundary of the original injury and it often occurs in areas of high motion. The hypertrophic scar develops earlier than the keloid, at less than 4 weeks after injury; it is more responsive to intervention including surgical excision and more likely to subside with time. An additional chapter in this volume discusses scarring in ethnic populations, including keloidal and hypertrophic scars, in greater depth.

Disease-related scars arising from acute inflammatory processes, such acne vulgaris or varicella zoster, often present as atrophic scars. These scars appear concave and the overlying skin can be paper-thin, as the associated inflammation results in collagen destruction with dermal atrophy. Acne scars can be further categorized clinically as ice pick, rolling, and boxcar scars. Ice pick scars are deep punctate scars while boxcar scars are shallow or deep, flat crateriform depressions in the skin. Rolling scars appear as irregular tethering of the skin, resulting in an uneven superficially wrinkled texture. Ice pick and deep boxcar scars respond well to punch excision, while rolling scars are best treated with subcision, fillers, or lasers. Punch elevation may also be used for wider, deep boxcar scars (> 3 mm).

## Patient Selection

In theory, any scar with a suboptimal appearance can be revised; however the greatest patient satisfaction can only be achieved with realistic expectations. Preoperative consultation should strive to educate and emphasize to the patient that a scar can never be completely removed but only exchanged for a more cosmetically pleasing one.

A number of considerations should be made before attempting a scar revision. A comprehensive patient medical history including response to past surgical procedures should be obtained. Certain patient populations, such as Asians, Hispanics, and black-skinned individuals, are predisposed to developing keloids and hypertrophic scars. Age also plays a factor, as the highest incidence of keloid development occurs between the ages of 10 and 30 years. Further caution should be exercised in patients with genetic disorders including Ehlers–Danlos and Marfan syndromes, endocrine abnormalities of the hypothalamus, thyroid, and parathyroid glands, or a history of radiation. Any of these conditions may result in an insufficient response to revision and subsequent poor scarring.

## Overview of Treatment Strategy

### General treatment approach

Prevention of a suboptimal scar is the best approach. Complete restoration of a scar to its preinjured state is impossible but careful preoperative planning will significantly reduce the need for future revision. However, timing is also important. While it can never be too late to revise a scar, it can be too early, as revisions done too early in the healing process can actually weaken the closure or lead to hypertrophy.

The surgical strategy selected should be based on a careful evaluation of the scar's characteristics: color, texture, type and timing of previous therapy, position and orientation, size, thickness, and quality of the surrounding skin. Special caution should be exercised with 'difficult' scars such as those that result from injuries where skin was lost from avulsion, necrosis, or large excisions, as skin laxity will be significantly diminished. The revision should be planned close to the original scar but not at the edge or margin of the scar.

Preoperative instructions for patients should include the avoidance of anticoagulant medications as medically appropriate including voluntary aspirin, nonsteroidal anti-inflammatory drugs (NSAIDs), vitamins C and E supplements, and alcohol for at least 1 week. Prophylactic antibiotics against wound infection should also be prescribed when indicated, such as for high-risk surgical sites (e.g. the axilla, perineum, and sites of cartilage exposure) or predisposing medical conditions (e.g. within 2 years after joint or valve replacement or immunosuppression).

## General Surgical Principles

Use a marking pen to outline planned incisions with the patient in an upright position prior to infiltration of local anesthetic. Be sure to mark or redefine key anatomic landmarks that may become obscured during surgery (e.g. vermillion border or nasolabial fold). During preoperative planning, an M-plasty can be utilized when it is necessary to respect anatomic landmarks, borders of cosmetic units, or shorten scars.

All procedures described in this chapter are performed under local anesthesia. The authors use 1% lidocaine with 1:100,000 epinephrine for a vasoconstrictive effect in areas with good collateral circulation. The surgical site should undergo sterile prep and drape. A

Bard-Parker No. 15 scalpel blade is generally used for excisional surgery.

Wounds heal best with clean, fresh, healthy edges; this can be achieved by approximating edges with minimal tension in the correct orientation and with the least reactive suture material selected. The authors employ buried vertical mattress sutures to minimize retraction of the subdermis and to displace tension off the healing wound edge. A well-placed buried vertical mattress suture as demonstrated in Figure 3.3 also yields tissue eversion. Suspension sutures to anchor the advancing tissue edge to periosteum can be employed to decrease tension on a free tissue margin such as the lip or eyelid and to recreate a natural fold or concavity.

For subcutaneous (SC) or dermal closures in areas of higher tension such as the trunk or extremities, the authors recommend an absorbable 4-0 suture. In sites of less tension such as the face, an absorbable 5-0 suture can be used for dermal closure. For cuticular closure, a non-absorbable 4-0 suture on the trunk or extremities can be employed, especially polypropylene for running intradermal sutures to reduce suture track marks. A nonabsorbable 5-0 or 6-0 suture on the face. Sutures can be left for 2 weeks on the trunk, although they can remain for longer periods of time if running intradermally or at sites of high tension. Generally sutures can be left on the face for 1 week. Fewer, although sufficient, deep sutures are better, as additional sutures increase the inflammatory response.

Postoperative care is critical to achieving a successful scar revision and relies on several key points. The authors use a pressure dressing for 24 hours postoperatively to encourage hemostasis. Patients are counseled to minimize sun exposure as well as trauma and tension to the scar site for as long as possible. They recommend an ointment such as Aquaphor Healing Ointment (Beiersdorf Inc., Wilton, CT) and a bandage for occlusion for 1 week on the face and 2 weeks on the

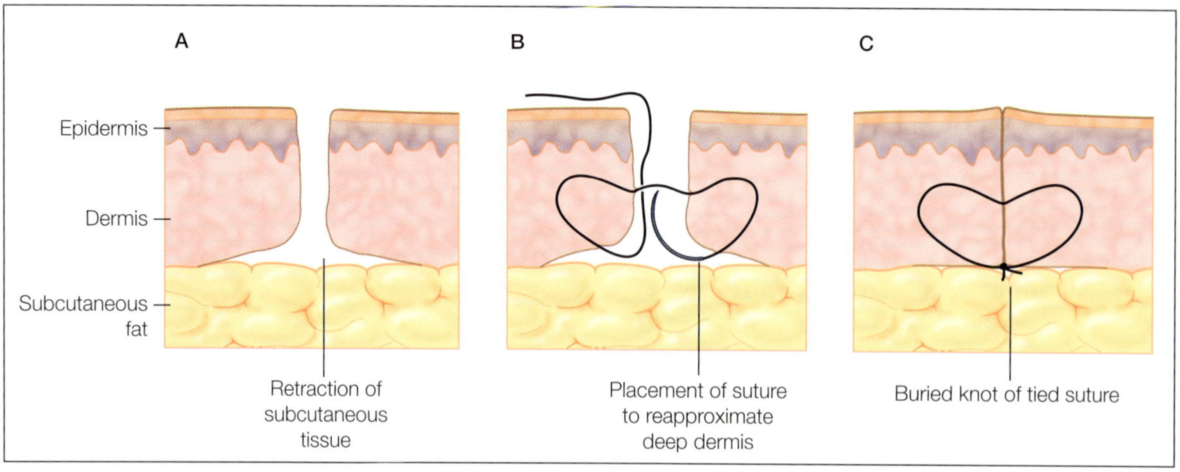


**Fig. 3.3** Buried vertical mattress stitch. (**A**) Retracted SC tissue after undermining. (**B**) Placement of buried vertical mattress suture. (**C**) Resultant wound edge eversion

trunk. Laser resurfacing or dermabrasion may follow 6–8 weeks postoperatively to further correct the appearance of the revised scar, if necessary.

## Treatment Techniques

### Excisional techniques

#### *Shave excision*

##### Indications

Shave excision is recommended for small standing cutaneous deformities and narrow scars with raised or uneven edges.

##### Treatment algorithm

Tangentially shave the scar with a flexible razor blade/scalpel until it is level with the surrounding skin, but avoid entry into deep dermis. If using a scalpel, it is often helpful to score the periphery of the elevated scar first to ensure that treatment does not extend beyond the intended area. Fine electrosurgery can be used to smooth the transition from the scar to surrounding skin, although this is not advised when shaving keloids. Allow the wound to heal by secondary intention.

#### *Fusiform excision*

Also known as **elliptical** or **extramarginal scar excision**, this technique leaves a fine linear scar in the natural creases of RSTLs.

##### Indications

Fusiform excision is very versatile and can be applied to revise anything from small (< 2 cm) scars that lie within RSTLs to medium-large scars, although they may require a series of excisions at 6–8-week intervals. Candidate scars for this procedure can be wide, depressed, or raised.

##### Treatment algorithm

Regardless of width and depth, aim for complete removal of scar tissue. As the name implies, the scar is removed as the center of an ellipse with opposing angles of 30 degrees or less. Adequate undermining is necessary to produce wound edges in an even and tension-free manner for a healthy healing environment. Fusiform excisions are demonstrated in Figures 3.4 and 3.5, and in an accompanying video clip.

##### Troubleshooting

**Deep defects.** Deeper and more extensive defects can also benefit from this technique, although they require more structural support upon removal of the scar. This can be achieved by creating a base with the first layer of sutures; an interrupted, simple absorbable suture works well in this situation. Good dermal approximation is realized with buried vertical mattress sutures, followed by simple interrupted

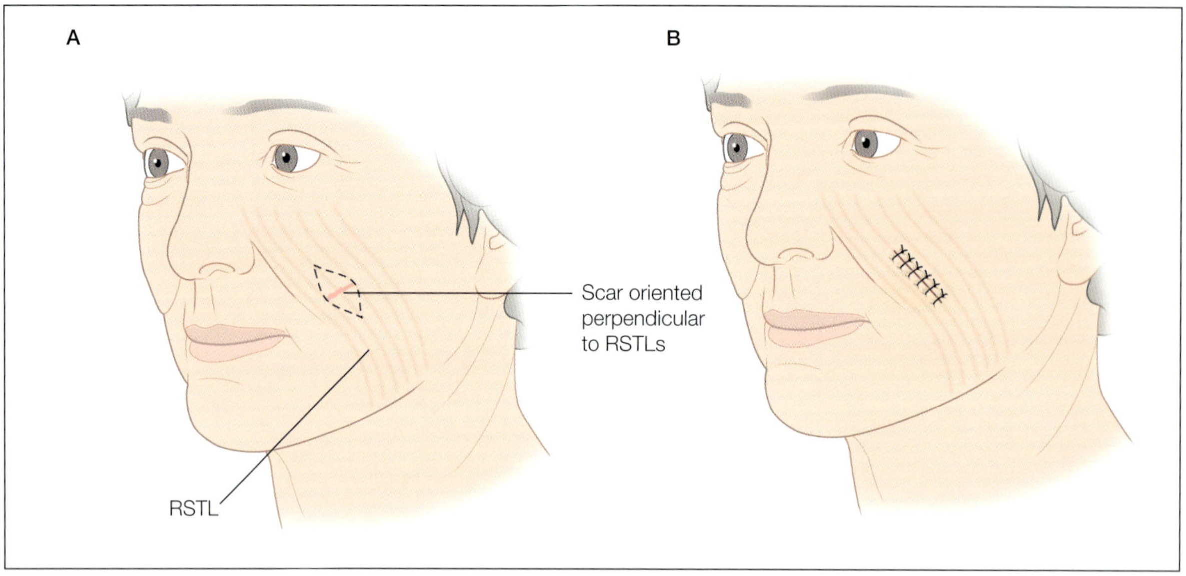


**Fig. 3.4** (**A** and **B**) Schematic of fusiform excision. Note reorientation of scar to within RSTLs

sutures or subcuticular stitches. A subcuticular approach is preferred for nonfacial areas because it leaves no punctate or cross-tie scars when sutures are left for longer than 1 week.

**Keloids and hypertrophic scars.** Avoid areas of high tension when revising keloid scars as they have a very high rate of recurrence (50–80%). Excise all potential sources of persistent inflammation, including epithelial cysts, sinus tracts, or any trapped hair follicles. The overlying uninvolved epidermis and upper dermis can be used as a source for a flap or graft by dissecting out the underlying keloidal collagen and replacing the upper dermis and epidermis over the site. With this technique, avoid SC sutures to prevent a subsequent inflammatory reaction and use epidermal sutures only.

## *Serial partial excision*

### Indications

This technique is especially valuable when the size and elasticity of the scar and surrounding skin prevents closure without distorting nearby structures.

### Treatment algorithm

Using conventional excision methods, partially excise the scar and advance the adjacent skin by undermining sufficiently. The number of required procedures depends on the size and location of the scar, as well as the relative elasticity of the surrounding skin. If more than two procedures are required, consider tissue expansion as a complementary tool to reduce the number of necessary excisions.

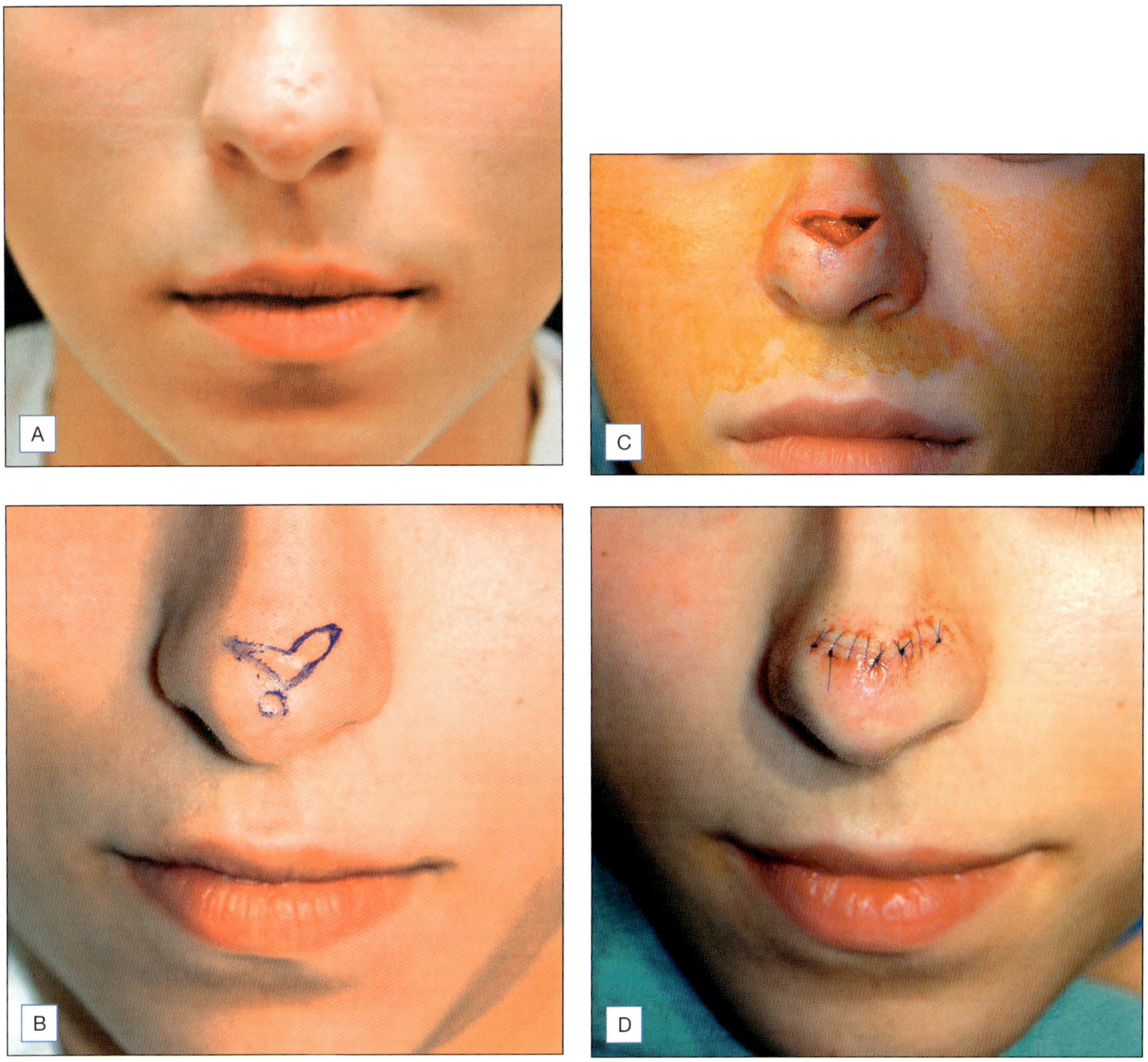

**Fig. 3.5** Clinical photos demonstrating fusiform excision technique. (**A**) Preoperative appearance of atrophic scars from trauma on dorsal aspect of nose. (**B**) Planned incision to remove scars. (**C**) Intraoperative photo after scars excised. (**D**) Revised scar after suture placement. Note eversion yielded by buried vertical mattress sutures

## Scar irregularization

Scar irregularization is especially beneficial in cases of elongated scars that cross anatomic subunits, distort anatomy, or are webbed. Scar irregularization is also beneficial to decrease the conspicuousness of long linear scars.

### *Z-plasty*

This technique diffuses forces and contractile distortion by transposing triangular skin flaps, changing the direction of the scar to lie within RSTLs.

## Indications

The Z-plasty has many uses, as it can lengthen a contracted scar, erase webs and clefts, reposition facial landmarks, provide hair camouflage, and break up long, straight scars (although other irregularization techniques can camouflage more effectively).

## Treatment algorithm

Mark lateral limb lengths before excising the scar. Removal of the main portion of scar creates the central limb and triangular flaps are cut to the same length as the central limb, although they may need to be lengthened depending on skin laxity. The final position of the central limb on the new 'Z' can be predicted by connecting the two free ends of the original Z (Fig. 3.6). The amount of lengthening depends on the angles of the limbs; a general rule of lengthening is that for each 15-degree angle change, the scar lengthens 25% (Table 3.3). The final

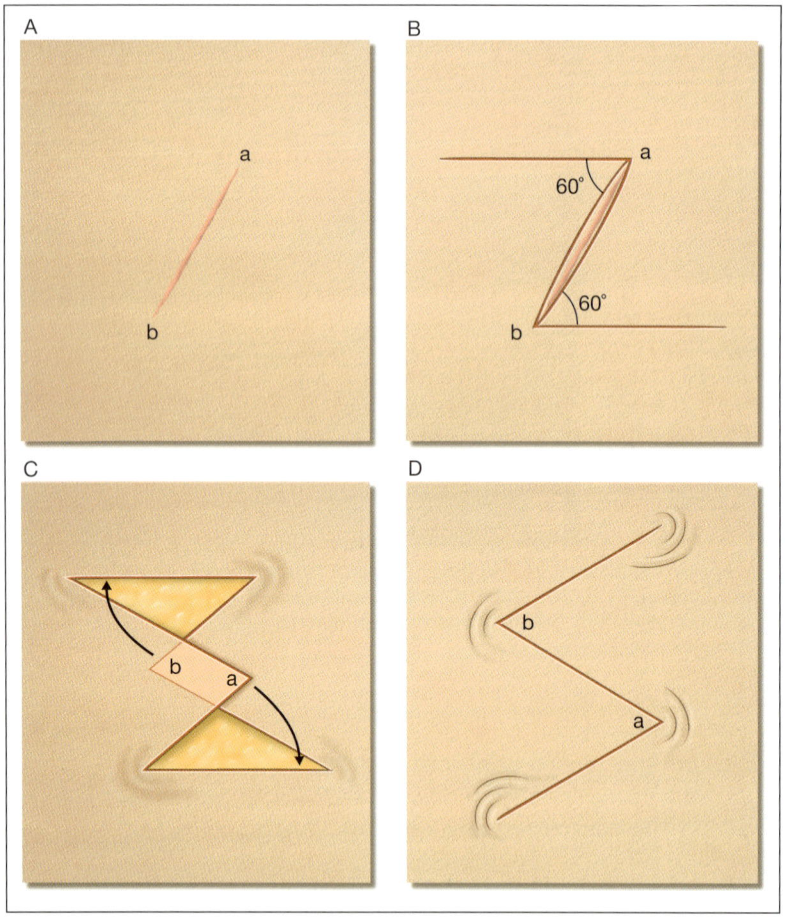


**Fig. 3.6** Z-plasty. Two additional limbs equal in length to the scar and parallel to RSTLs are used to create transposition flaps. (**A**) Scar oriented A–B. (**B**) Scar excised and creation of flaps with two limbs parallel to RSTLs. A 60-degree angle will yield a 75% increase in wound length. (**C**) Movement of the flaps. (**D**) Resultant scar with reorientation of **A–B**

scar will be approximately three times longer than the original scar, and multiple Z-plasties can be combined in series to reduce tissue contraction (Fig. 3.7). The surrounding tissue is undermined, and the two triangles are then transposed. It is important to properly release the flaps to allow the tips to have little tension and avoid tip necrosis.

#### Contraindications

Avoid in keloid reconstruction since a keloid may form along the lengthened scar line and be worse than the original problem.

| Z-Plasty Predicted Net Tissue Gain | |
|---|---|
| **Angle of Z-plasty (degrees)** | **Percent tissue gain** |
| 30 | 25 |
| 45 | 50 |
| 60 | 75 |

**Table 3.3** Z-plasty predicted net tissue gain

### *W-plasty*

The advantage of this technique stems from the fact that it does not lengthen the scar. Although its pattern is more predictable and therefore less camouflaging than the revision achieved by geometric broken line closure, it is a faster procedure.

#### Indications

A W-plasty may be used for long, straight scars (> 2 cm) that are perpendicular to RSTLs and traverse convex curvature areas such as the mandibular border, cheek, or forehead. It is also helpful for contracted scars and short scars on the forehead or neck.

#### Treatment algorithm

Careful preplanning is essential, as a series of small interdigitating triangular skin flaps (several small 'Ws') are positioned on either side of the original scar so that the two sides will interpose perfectly after scar excision and local undermining. Triangle limbs should be 3–5 mm long and ends should be less than 30 degrees in order to avoid a standing cone or 'dog ear' effect. Components should parallel RSTLs as much as possible to provide optimal camouflage. Scar tissue should be completely excised and undermined widely for a tension-free closure (Fig. 3.8). The W-plasty technique can also be used to camouflage curvilinear scars (Fig. 3.9).

#### Contraindications

In areas with little skin laxity, closure can be problematic.

### *Geometric broken-line closure*

Geometric broken-line closure (GBLC) is the most sophisticated scar irregularization technique, providing better camouflage (irregular irregularity) without scar lengthening, but it takes longer to perform and is more technically challenging.

#### Indications

Like the W-plasty, this technique works best for long, straight scars that traverse or are perpendicular to RSTLs.

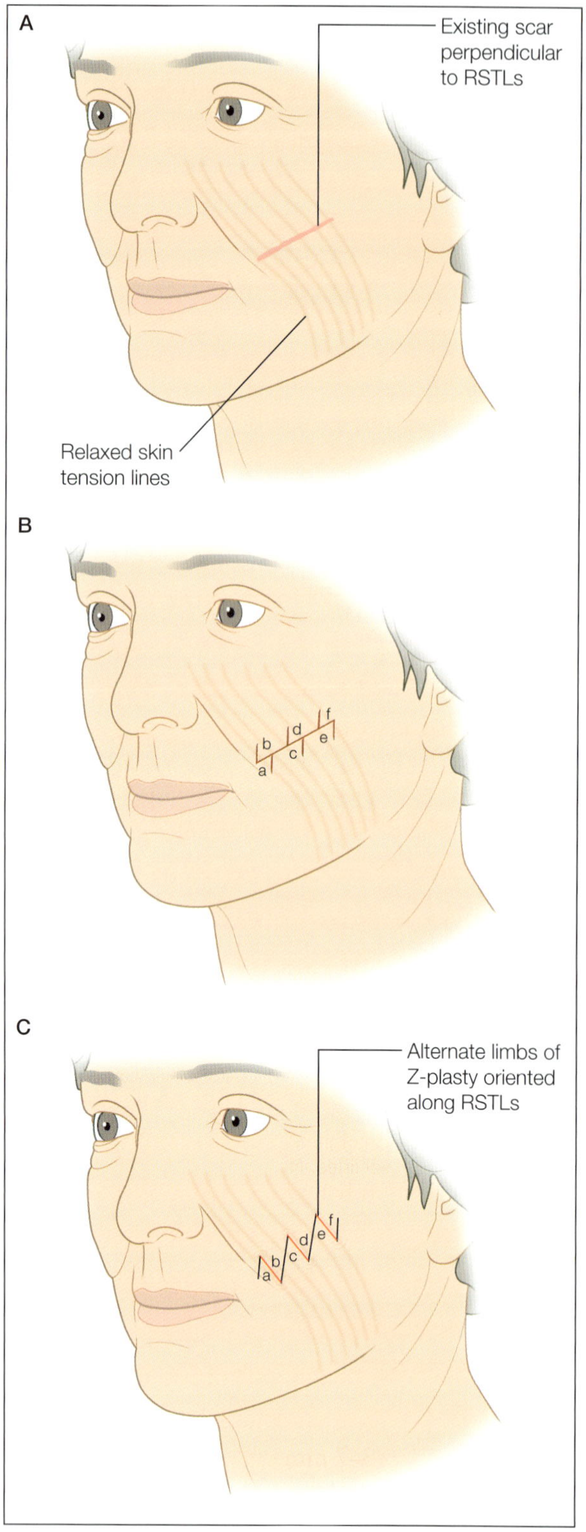


**Fig. 3.7** Series of Z-plasties. (**A**) Long scar oriented against relaxed skin tension lines (RSTLs). (**B**) Creation of multiple Z-plasty flaps. a and b are interposed, c and d are interposed, and e and f are interposed. (**C**) Resultant scar with alternate limbs highlighted in red oriented along RSTLs

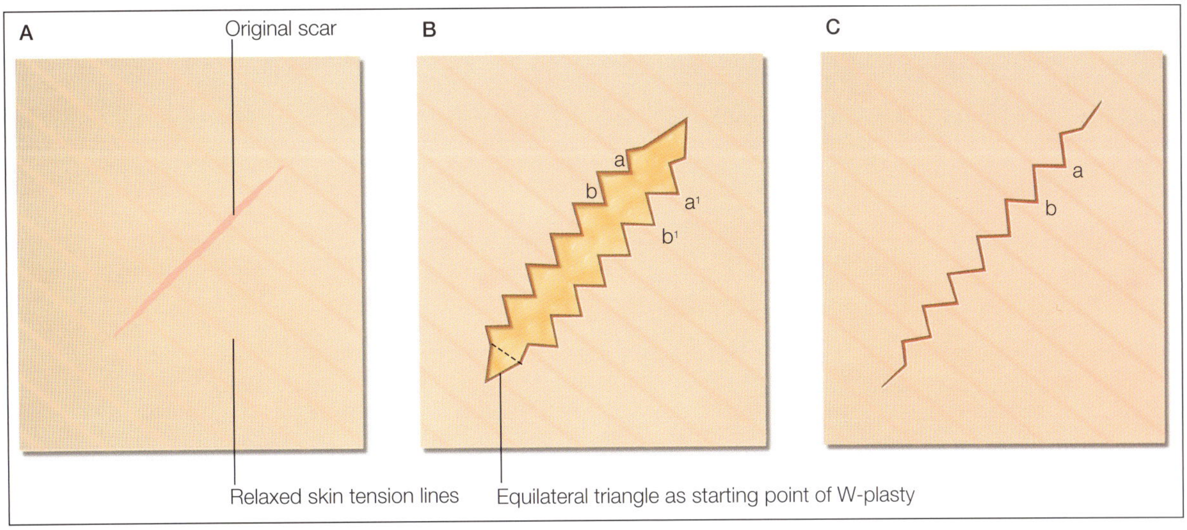


**Fig. 3.8** W-plasty. (**A**) Straight line scar. (**B**) Irregularization with a pattern of interdigitating Ws positioned on either side of the wound. Note correspondence of points a and $a^1$ and b and $b^1$. (**C**) Interposition of the Ws after scar excision with a resultant zig-zag line in which half of the lines are oriented along RSTLs. Note resulting positions of a and b

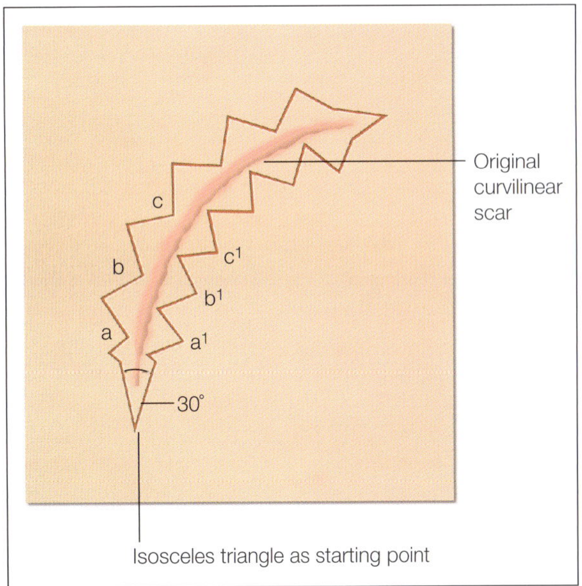


**Fig. 3.9** W-plasty revision of a curvilinear scar. Use of a 30-degree isosceles triangle as a starting point for complimentary parallel lines. Note that the angles of the inner incision are more acute but the lengths of the sides are roughly the same as those of the outer incision. This allows point a to correspond to $a^1$ and b to $b^1$ etc.

## Treatment algorithm

Rather than employing 'Ws,' the GBLC involves a series of varying geometric shapes designed to interlock precisely with their mirror images on the other side of the wound. Geometric shapes should vary irregularly and be 3–7 mm in size placed 3–6 mm from the scar margin (Fig. 3.10). The treatment area should be undermined widely for a tension-free closure, although the deeper portion of the old scar should not be excised. As was the case in the W-plasty, ends should be less than 30 degrees or an M-plasty should be used to avoid dog ears.

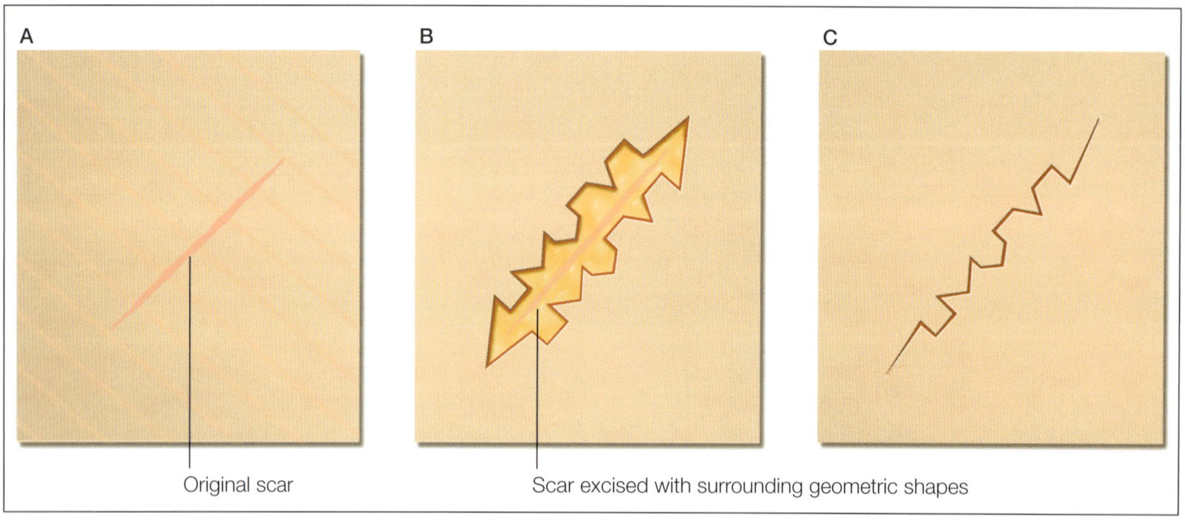


**Fig. 3.10** GBLC. (**A**) Scar. (**B**) Irregularly irregular lock-in-key design of geometric shapes. Although figure is enlarged for detail, shapes should be between 5–7 mm each. Sharp-angled shapes are less perceptible than circles or ovals in the final scar result. (**C**) Irregular final result minimizes perceptibility of scar

## Acne/Atrophic Scar Revision

The appropriateness and efficacy of the following techniques depends highly on the type of atrophic scar being revised.

### Subcision

This procedure is based on the physiology of rolling scars, releasing the SC fibrotic strands that pull down the overlying tissue. The controlled trauma creates new connective tissue formation under the defect for additional support. Collagen formation continues for months after the procedure, and at 12 months after the procedure, patients and physicians rate up to a 50% improvement in the appearance of rolling scars with this technique. Fillers, discussed later, may be used following subcision to improve the appearance of remaining depressed scars.

#### *Indications*

This technique works best for rolling acne scars and other scars that improve with the stretching of skin during examination.

#### *Treatment algorithm*

Insert a sterile 18 gauge, 1½ inch Nokor Admix needle (Becton Dickinson and Co., Franklin Lakes, NJ) on a 3 cc syringe at a shallow angle, with the blade situated parallel to the skin surface. The needle should be inserted into the superficial SC layer, and occasionally, into the deep dermis. The free hand should be used to stabilize the site while the needle moves in a lancing and fanning motion to release

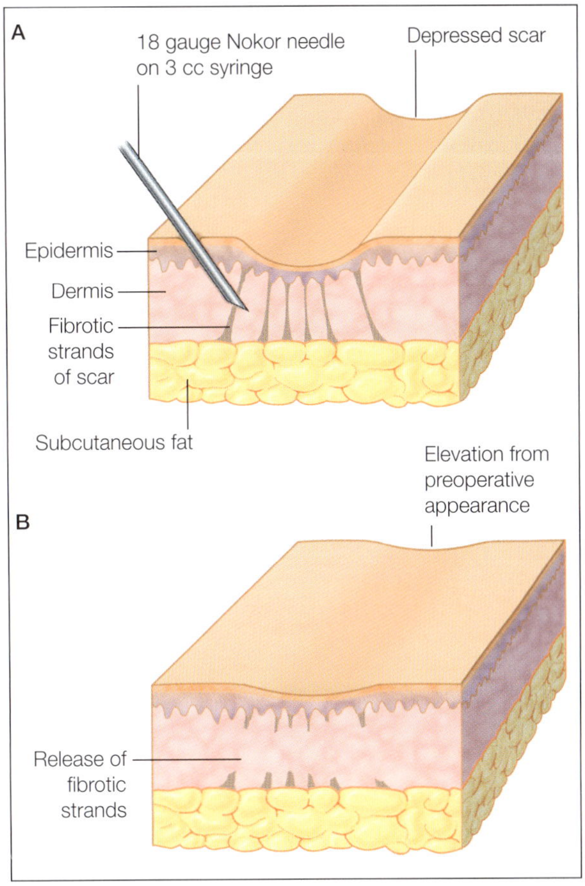


**Fig. 3.11** Subcision for rolling acne scar. **(A)** Needle inserted at acute angle with blade oriented parallel to skin surface. Needle used to break up fibrous strands of scar. **(B)** Scar smoother and elevated from preoperative tethered appearance

the SC fibrotic strands (Fig. 3.11). For maximal release of the fibrotic strands, it is best to approach the scar from multiple puncture sites. Firm pressure should be applied postoperatively for at least 5 minutes to achieve hemostasis. For severe rolling scars or extensive areas of involvement, subcision can be repeated at 6-week intervals for up to three successive treatments.

### *Troubleshooting*

Hematomas, hypertrophic scarring, and scar recurrence are side effects associated with this procedure. If a hypertrophic scar does develop during healing, inject intralesional triamcinolone 3.3–10 mg/cc as indicated by the scar firmness until the site flattens. The risk of side effects increases with multiple subcision sessions.

## Punch excision

### *Indications*

Punch excision is recommended for revising icepick or deep boxcar scars.

### *Treatment algorithm*

When planning the excision, use outward traction perpendicular to RSTLs so that the circular wound becomes an ellipse and closes parallel to RSTLs (Fig. 3.12). Depending on the size of the scar, a 1.5–3 mm punch can be used to remove the entire defect.

## Punch elevation

The stated advantage of this procedure over punch grafting is the avoidance of color or texture mismatch; however, because scar tissue is being used, color and textural irregularities may persist.

### *Indications*

Punch elevation works best for wide (> 3 mm) boxcar acne scars that do not have significant color or textural irregularities.

### *Treatment algorithm*

Match the punch size to the inner diameter of the crateriform scar. Punch using a quick, rotating motion to release the bound-down scar and elevate with forceps so that the scar lies slightly higher than the surrounding skin. Free the plug from underlying tissue and secure with Dermabond (2-Octyl Cyanoacrylate, Ethicon Inc., Somerville, NJ) and paper tape such as Steri-Strips (3M Corp., St Paul, MN).

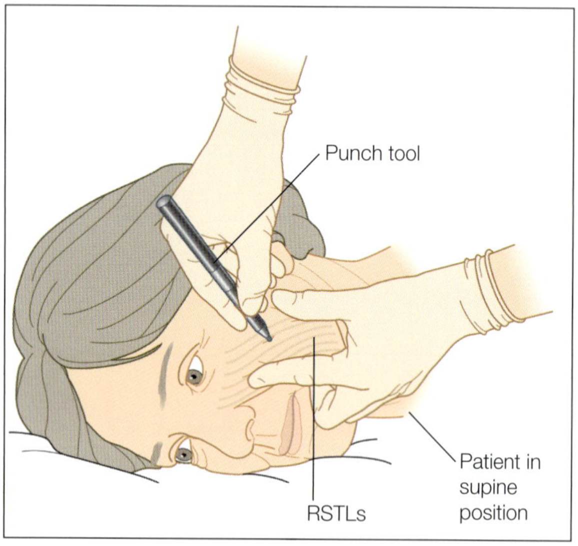


**Fig. 3.12** Schematic of technique for punch excision. Note use of nondominant hand to apply outward traction perpendicular to RSTLs. The punch tool is placed perpendicular to the skin and used with a quick rotating motion to remove the scar

## Punch grafting

Given the number of possible complications associated with this procedure, punch grafting is recommended only as second-line therapy.

### *Indications*

Deep, irregular scars or tethered boxcar scars benefit from this technique, which works best on less mobile areas of the face such as the forehead, but not as well in dynamic areas, such as the perioral sites.

### *Treatment algorithm*

This technique is similar to punch elevation, but replaces the plug with a donor plug instead of elevating the original defect. After excising the scar, a graft that is equal in size or up to 0.5 mm larger than the original plug is taken from the postauricular donor site and placed in the recipient site. The donor site is sutured and the recipient site is secured with Dermabond (2-Octyl Cyanoacrylate, Ethicon Inc., Somerville, NJ) and paper tape such as Steri-Strips (3M Corp., St Paul, MN).

### *Troubleshooting*

Postoperative sequelae include poor graft take, graft extrusion, and graft visibility due to mismatch of graft color or texture.

## Fillers

### Indications

Fillers are best used for sauceriform acne scars, concave defects with the dermis, or easily distensible scars. The more mature and supple the scar, the better the results. Due to the localized trauma from injection of any filler, the body produces some collagen; therefore, scars treated with fillers become less deep after the first injection. Ice pick scars and postvaricella scars do not respond well to this treatment because they tend to have a significant epidermal component to them. The position of a dermal filler is demonstrated in Figure 3.13.

### Types of fillers

#### *Injectables*

Collagen is injected into the site with a 30 gauge needle, bevel up. Bovine collagen (e.g. Zyplast, Zyderm, Inamed Corp., Santa Barbara, CA) requires skin testing, as 3.5% of patients have a positive delayed type skin reaction. Correction varies from 3–18 months, but patients with a history of autoimmune disease should be excluded. Human collagen (e.g. Cosmoplast, Cosmoderm, Inamed Corp., Santa Barbara, CA) can also be used, as allergic reactions are less common, but the effect is shorter and usually lasts only 3–4 months. Another option is hyaluronic acid, which also does not require allergy testing and lasts longer than human collagen, at least 6–8 months. Hyaluronic acid is available as Restylane (Medicis Aesthetics, Scottsdale, AZ; Q-Med

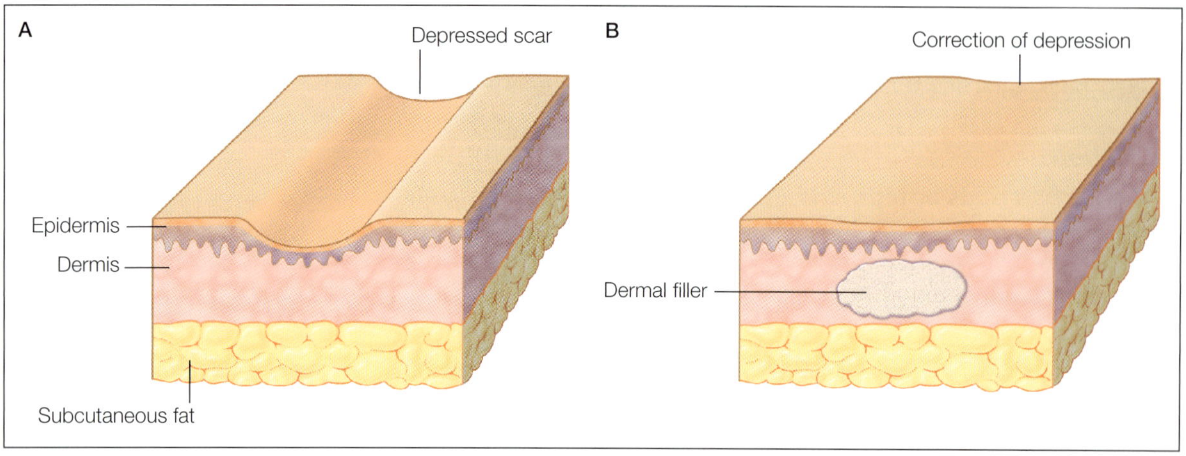


**Fig. 3.13** Position of dermal filler for depressed scar

Laboratories, Uppsala, Sweden), Hylaform or Captique (both Inamed Corp., Santa Barbara, CA). Hyaluronic acid products currently under FDA review in the United States include Perlane (Medicis Aesthetics, Scottsdale, AZ; Q-Med Laboratories, Uppsala, Sweden) and Juvederm (Euromedical Systems Ltd., Nottingham, England).

Fillers which include particles to stimulate greater fibrosis may be longer lasting. Several of these fillers at the time of this publication are not yet FDA approved in the United States or their use for scars may be off label. These fillers are injected in small amounts in the deep dermis to avoid beading and to incite surrounding fibrosis. Longer lasting fillers include polymethylmethacrylate microspheres with partly denatured bovine collagen (Artecoll and Artefill, Artes Medical Inc., San Diego, CA), poly-L-lactic acid (Sculptra Dermik Aesthetics, Aventis Pharmaceuticals, Bridgewater, NJ), calcium hydroxyapatite (Radiance, Bioform, Inc., San Mateo, CA) and medical grade silicone (Silikon 1000, Alcon Laboratories Inc., Fort Worth, TX).

Newer fillers derived from human skin attempt to reconstruct the dermal matrix. At the time of this publication, these modalities are not yet FDA approved for use on scars. Collagen harvested from the patient is cultured for fibroblasts by a biotechnology company and then returned for serial injections into the patient as Autologen (Collagenesis Inc., Beverly, MA) or Isolagen (Isolagen Inc., Houston, TX). Acellular human cadaveric dermis is available in a freeze-dried or in an injectable, micronized form, respectively as Alloderm and Cymetra (LifeCell Corp., Branchburg, NJ). Contraindications to the use of acellular dermal matrix include an allergy to gentamicin, a history of collagen vascular disease, and a poorly vascularized recipient site.

For deep defects, implantable fillers may achieve longer lasting correction but may have a higher risk of complications including infection and extrusion. These include expanded polytetrafluoroethylene such as Gore-Tex (W.L. Gore and Associates, Flagstaff, AZ) or SoftForm (Tissue Technologies Inc., San Francisco, CA).

## Fat Transplantation

This technique requires special equipment and training and has variable longevity, as an average of 50% of the transplanted fat can be resorbed after 1 year. Blood-free, yellow adipose tissue is transferred into 3 cc syringes and the lipoinjection is performed using a 16–18 gauge needle. The tool is advanced into the scar and the adipose tissue is injected as the needle is withdrawn. This process continues until a 100% correction is achieved. Scarring is uncommon and repeat injections may be conducted at 6–12-week intervals. Overcorrection may yield bumps or textural irregularities after incomplete resorption.

## Dermal Grafting

This technique builds on subcision to place permanent retroauricular dermal grafts into precise pockets under the skin. Although the end result is dependent on technique, there are theoretical advantages associated with these grafts as they are readily available, not susceptible to rejection, create a permanent spacer between the overlying skin and the underlying fibrous band of scar tissue, and can be accurately tailored for a variety of defects.

The scar is undermined 10–14 days before the operation with an 18 gauge needle in order to stimulate granulation tissue and achieve some initial correction. The donor site for the dermis is usually hidden in the retroauricular sulcus or neck. After the epidermis of this donor site is removed using dermabrasion, $CO_2$ laser, or scalpel, the dermis is harvested down to the deep fascia level with 3 mm punches or long narrow strips, defatted, and placed in saline. The harvested dermis is shaped to fit the site of the scar and placed in the previously created pocket within and under the scar with a stab incision. An epidermal suture can be used to close the pocket. A schematic of the dermal grafting technique is shown in Figure 3.14.

## Dermabrasion

Early intervention with this method yields optimal results, but it is a highly technique-dependent procedure. Lasers are now used more commonly than dermabrasion for postoperative resurfacing. The use of lasers is discussed in depth in a separate chapter of this volume.

### Indications

While dermabrasion can be used for isolated lesions (acne, pox, trapdoor) and raised scars, it is more commonly employed as a secondary procedure 6–8 weeks after scar revision and is useful for smoothing skin surface contour irregularities.

### Treatment algorithm

Begin retinoic acid or hydroquinone 4% 1 month in advance to encourage re-epithelialization and decrease the risk of post-inflammatory

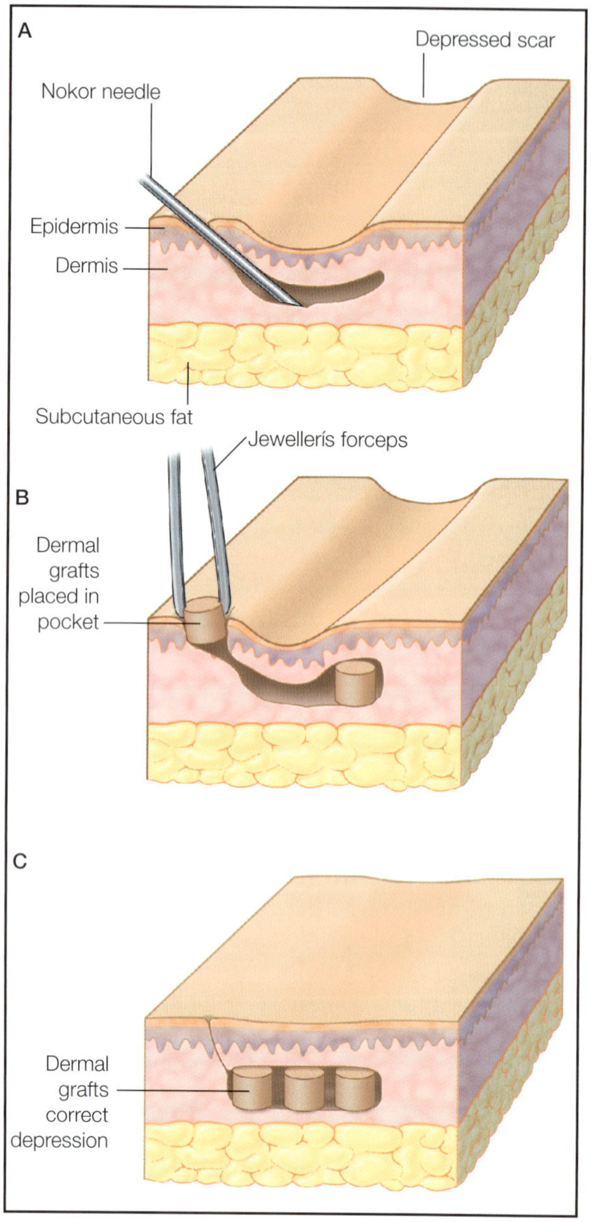


**Fig. 3.14** Dermal grafting. (**A**) Depressed scar is undermined with 18 gauge, 1.5 in Nokor Admix needle (Becton Dickinson and Co., Franklin Lakes, NJ) approximately 2 weeks before dermal graft procedure. Undermining stimulates granulation tissue and initiates collagenesis. Subcision with Nokor needle is repeated to create a pocket for dermal grafts on day of procedure. (**B**) Dermal grafts are inserted into pocket with jeweler's forceps. (**C**) Correction of depression with grafts in place

hyperpigmentation, respectively. Because particles can become airborne and aerosolized during this procedure, all operating room staff should take appropriate safety precautions. Local anesthesia (tumescent or refrigerant agents) will produce a firm surface without distorting the skin. Care should be taken to keep the treatment area free of any materials that may interfere with the dermabrader (e.g. hair, towels, gauze).

The dermabrader is a motor-driven handpiece (20,000 to 30,000 r.p.m.) with an attached diamond fraise that can vary from fine to coarse. It should be held at 90 degrees to the direction of wheel rotation and advanced in the direction of wheel rotation. The scar should be rapidly sculpted, aiming for mid-papillary or deep papillary dermis penetration, as the reticular dermis and adnexal structures must be preserved in order to re-epithelialize without scarring. Make sure to feather the periphery of the dermabraded area to produce a smooth transition between treated and untreated areas. Iced gauze will stop any remaining bleeding. Patients will re-epithelialize within 5–7 days, although erythema lasting 2–3 months is normal.

### Contraindications

Avoid patients with active herpetic lesions or who have been treated with isotretinoin within the preceding year. This procedure also carries a risk of post-inflammatory pigmentary alteration.

## Dermasanding (Manual Dermabrasion)

### Indications

Dermasanding can be used for the same indications as dermabrasion. It is a simpler, less expensive, and safer procedure without the blood splatter or aerosolized potentially infectious particles of dermabrasion.

### Treatment algorithm

Sterile strips of waterproof silicone carbide sandpaper are used to gently abrade the scar. Sandpaper strips can be wrapped around the finger or the barrel of a 3 cc syringe to provide a firm platform. Start with 200 grit sandpaper until pinpoint bleeding is observed, then smooth with 400 grit sandpaper. Hemostasis is achieved with topical 1% lidocaine with epinephrine and pressure. Sandpaper dermabrasion is demonstrated in Figure 3.15. Postinflammatory hyperpigmentation may develop, but will resolve with time. Pre- and postoperative topical hydroquinone may minimize this risk.

## Conclusion

As can be gleaned from this chapter, numerous surgical techniques are available for scar revision. While some are better suited to treat specific types of scars, they can be used in combination with each other or with other scar revision techniques to achieve optimal results. A clear knowledge of basic surgical revision techniques can be applied to help patients achieve more aesthetically pleasing scars in the most predictable and efficacious manner.

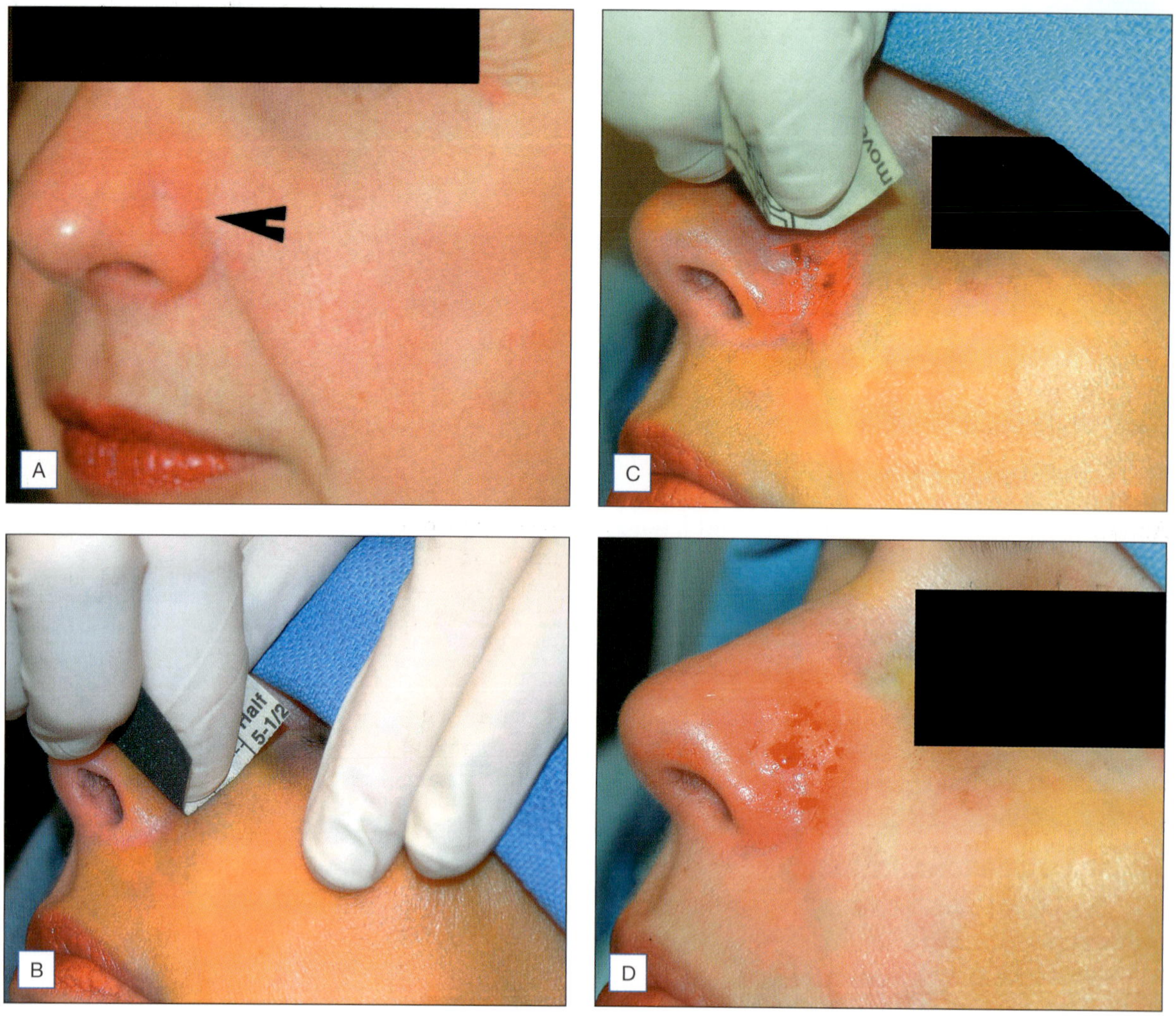


**Fig. 3.15** Clinical photos demonstrating sandpaper dermabrasion to correct scar contour. (**A**) Preoperative raised scar on nasal sidewall (*arrowhead*). (**B**) Sanding technique. (**C**) Appearance of scar intraoperatively. (**D**) Scar appearance immediately after dermasanding. Note pinpoint bleeding

## Further Reading

Brodland D 1998 Complex closures. In: Ratz JL. Textbook of Dermatologic Surgery Philadelphia, Lippincott-Raven, pp 183–200

Gold MH 2003 Dermabrasion in dermatology. American Journal of Clinical Dermatology 4:467–471

Kaplan B, Potter T, Moy RL 1997 Scar revision. Dermatologic Surgery 23:435–442

McGillis ST, Lucas AR 1998 Scar revision. Dermatologic Clinics 16:165–180

Mostafapour SP, Murakami CS 2001 Tissue expansion and serial excision in scar revision. Facial Plastic Surgery 17:245–251

Poulous E, Taylor C, Solish N 2003 Effectiveness of dermasanding (manual dermabrasion) on the appearance of surgical scars: A prospective randomized, blinded study. Journal of the American Academy of Dermatology 48(6):897–900

Rodgers BJ, Williams EF, Hove CR 2001 W-Plasty and geometric broken line closure. Facial Plastic Surgery 17:239–244

Schweinfurth JM, Fedok F 2001 Avoiding pitfalls and unfavorable outcomes in scar revision. Facial Plastic Surgery 17(4):273–277

Swinehart JM 2001 Dermal grafting. Dermatologic Clinics 19(3):509–522

Thomas JR, Prendiville S 2002 Update in scar revision. Facial Plastic Surgery Clinics of North America 10:103–111

Tsao SS, Dover JS, Arndt KA, Kaminer MS 2002 Scar management: Keloid, hypertrophic, atrophic and acne scars. In: Kaminer MS, Dover JS, Arndt, KA (eds) Atlas of Cosmetic Surgery. Philadelphia: WB Saunders Co., pp 433–459

# 4 Treatment of Scars with Lasers and Other Energy Sources

*Keyvan Nouri, Maria Patricia Rivas, Christopher J. Ballard*

## Introduction

### The problem being treated

Almost all individuals in their lifetime will have a scar resulting from unexpected trauma, inflammation, burns or a surgical procedure involving incision of the skin. Irrespective of the cause of the scar, the wound healing process may result in either a 'normal' scar or in some other pathologic scar types such as hypertrophic, keloid, or atrophic scars.

Initially, normal scars appear erythematous and with an irregular surface; however, as the wound healing process continues, the mature scar acquires a skin-colored tone and its surface becomes more even and flat. Histology of normal scars shows hyalinized collagen lying parallel to the surface of the skin, with a decreased amount of elastic fibers.

Hypertrophic scars arise as red, raised firm scars that are limited to the incision or original injury site (Fig. 4.1). They are frequently linear, and a significant percentage of them are accompanied by sensation abnormalities such as pruritus. Hypertrophic scars usually appear

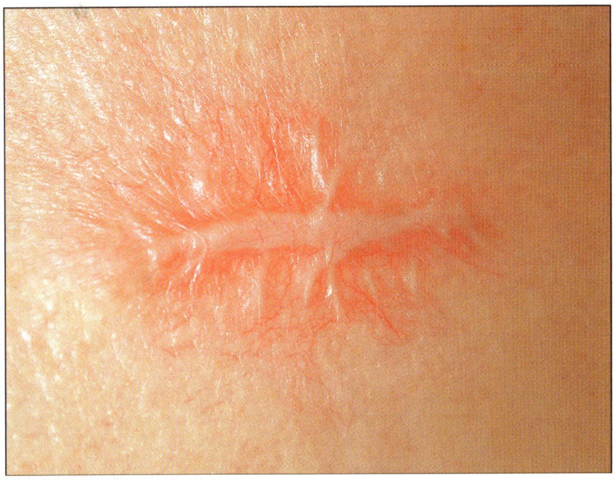

**Fig. 4.1** Hypertrophic scar: raised, erythematous scar, limited to the incision site

within 1 month of injury and may either continue to grow or involute with time. Hypertrophic scars may be located anywhere on the body; however those areas under constant pressure and stretching are more commonly affected.

Keloids are clinically described as purple nodules that extend beyond the original injury boundaries (Fig. 4.2), and can be associated to abnormal sensations. They are frequently disfiguring and may result in functional impairment. Keloids appear within weeks or years from original cutaneous insult. The most common locations for keloids are the earlobes, anterior chest, shoulders, and upper back. Besides the usual cutaneous injuries that cause scarring, keloids may also result from ear piercing, abrasions, tattooing, and vaccinations, among others. Complete resolution of keloids is very difficult as they do not spontaneously regress and have high recurrence rates, appearing even years later, with most therapies. There is a familial and ethnic predisposition to the formation of keloids, with darker skinned individuals having a higher incidence.

In contrast to hypertrophic scars and keloids, which result from excessive collagen deposition and scar tissue formation, atrophic scars, on the other hand, are the result of connective tissue destruction, with dermal atrophy and fibrosis.

Atrophic scars are commonly seen in patients with a history of acne (Fig. 4.3); however, other conditions such as varicella, surgery, and trauma may also result in atrophic scarring. Recently, a classification of acne scars into three types, namely icepick scars, rolling scars, and boxcar scars, has been proposed based on the scar's width, depth, and three-dimensional architecture. Icepick scars are seen as narrow

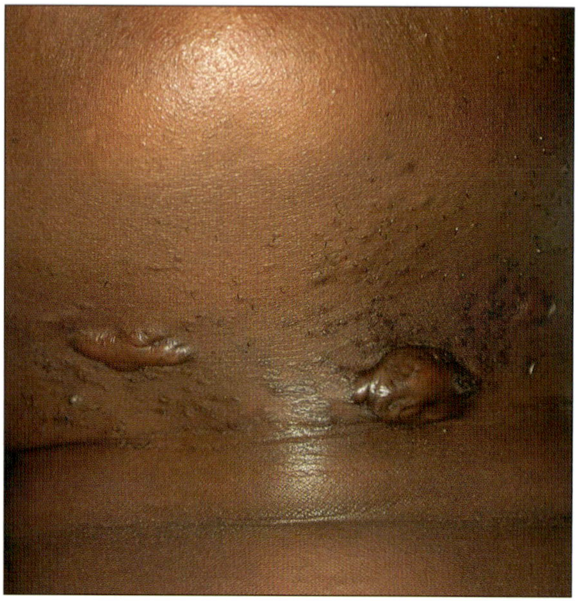

**Fig. 4.2** Keloid scars located on the neck of an African-American woman

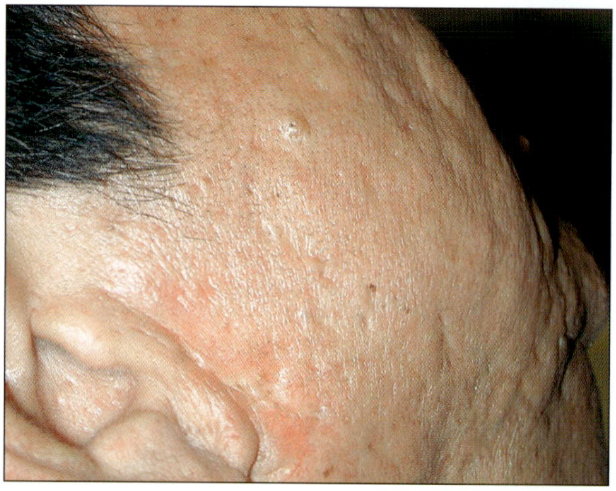

**Fig. 4.3** Adult male patient with post-acne atrophic facial scarring. The majority of the scars correspond to the icepick type. Some rolling-type scars can also be seen

and deep, their width decreasing as they extend into the dermis. Rolling scars have a wide surface with margins that give a 'rolling' appearance to the skin. Also with a wide surface, the boxcar scar type is limited by well-demarcated vertical borders.

The psychological burden of a scar, no matter which type, goes beyond the cosmetic appearance of it, and both patients and physicians alike are always seeking new scar revision alternatives that may further improve the outcome.

In general, and depending on the scar type, treatment options include surgery, cryotherapy, electrocautery and desiccation, dermabrasion, intralesional corticosteroids, 5-fluorouracil (5-FU), topical imiquimod, radiation, and lasers. Among the lasers that have been used for the treatment of scars are carbon dioxide ($CO_2$), erbium:yttrium-aluminum-garnet (Er:YAG), pulsed-dye laser (PDL), neodymium: yttrium-aluminum-garnet (Nd:YAG), and fractional resurfacing (Fraxel), among others (Table 4.1).

Over the years the above-mentioned different treatment options have been offered, some of which have dropped in popularity due to their side effects and poor outcome, whereas others are still used alone or in combination with others. Currently, the PDL is considered the laser of choice for the treatment of hypertrophic scars and keloids. Skin resurfacing with the $CO_2$ and Er:YAG lasers, as well as newer therapies such as the fractional resurfacing laser are being used for atrophic post-acne scarring. Plasma skin rejuvenation, a novel form of resurfacing/rejuvenation, will likely prove to be an effective method for modifying textural irregularities.

## Patient Selection

Patients with scars usually seek treatment due to their unfavorable cosmetic appearance, which may result in psychologic burden and

**Treatment Options According to the Type of Scar**

| Type of scar | Laser devices | Nonlaser treatments |
|---|---|---|
| Hypertrophic or keloid | Pulsed-dye laser<br>Q-switched Nd:YAG 532 nm | Intralesional 5-FU<br>Occlusion (silicone gel sheets)<br>Intralesional steroids<br>Topical imiquimod |
| Atrophic | Ablative lasers:<br>$CO_2$ laser<br>Er:YAG<br>Fractional resurfacing<br>Nonablative lasers:<br>Nd:YAG 1320 nm<br>Diode 1450 nm<br>Q-switched Nd:YAG 1064 nm<br>Erbium glass 1540 nm | Punch excision<br>Punch elevation<br>Subcision<br>Dermal fillers<br>Dermal grafting<br>Plasma resurfacing |

**Table 4.1** Treatment options according to the type of scar

social withdrawal. In addition, the presence of associated symptoms such as pruritus and dysesthesias, specifically in the patients with hypertrophic scars and keloids, may also incite the patient to seek medical attention.

Patient-specific factors such as skin type and lesion-specific factors such as age of scar, color, and number of lesions need to be considered when assessing therapeutic alternatives, such as lasers, for the treatment of scarring.

Skin tone is the main patient factor to be considered when thinking about scar revision with lasers. Skin tone has a great influence in the outcome of the treatment, with fair-skinned individuals having an overall better response, with fewer side effects such as pigmentation changes. When used in dark-skinned individuals, the epidermal melanin may compete for laser light absorption, which may result in reduced targeting of the lesion and skin pigmentation changes. Patients should be specifically notified about the high risk of pigmentation alterations that may result from laser treatment. In addition, some authors suggest using a test spot in an effort to anticipate any side effects and determine the most adequate parameter to be used. Many authors agree that when treating patients with skin types IV–VI, lower energies should be used, which may consequently result in the need of more treatment sessions to achieve the desired result.

Evaluation of the scar type, age and number of lesions is also necessary to determine eligibility for laser treatment. Hypertrophic scars that are relatively new, namely approximately less than 1 year old, that appear red are ideal for treatment with the PDL. In the case of atrophic scars, the number of lesions also needs to be evaluated. When only a few lesions are present, spot resurfacing may be considered, whereas for multiple scattered scars laser treatment of the entire cosmetic unit may be more adequate.

## Wound-healing Process

The wound-healing process is usually divided into three stages: (i) inflammation, (ii) proliferation, and (iii) remodeling. Once the injury has occurred, initiation of the inflammation phase occurs along with activation of the clotting and complement cascade. Chemotactic factors such as prostaglandins, complement factors, and interleukin-1 (IL-1) stimulate the migration of inflammatory cells such as neutrophils and macrophages. These cells initiate the debridement of the wound, and macrophages release cytokines and growth factors such as transforming growth factors (TGF-β), and platelet-derived growth factors (PDGFs), among others, leading to the formation of the provisional wound matrix. The migration of fibroblasts, endothelial cells, and keratinocytes to the wound site characterizes the unfolding of the proliferation stage. Fibroblasts play a major role in the formation of the extracellular matrix composed of collagen III and I, fibronectin, elastin, and proteoglycans. The keratinocytes start the re-epithelialization of the wound with reconstitution of the basement membrane. The presence of endothelial cells in the wound bed, stimulated by hypoxia and angiogenic factors such as FGF, results in the formation of new blood vessels. Remodeling of the collagen and proteoglycans takes place during the maturation phase. During this process hyaluronic acid is gradually replaced by glycosaminoglycans, such as chondroitine-sulfate and dermatan-sulfate. Both collagen types I and III increase during the wound healing process; however, as the scar continues to mature and remodeling takes place, the proportion of collagen type III decreases.

## Pathogenesis of Hypertrophic Scars and Keloids

Multiple disturbances in the wound healing process have been implicated in the development of hypertrophic scars and keloids; however, the precise mechanism has not been established. The development of excessive scar tissue seen in these types of pathologic scars may be due to either excessive matrix deposition, reduced collagen degradation, or both.

Fibroblasts from keloids show an abnormal response to stimulation, producing high levels of collagen, especially type I. On the other hand, fibroblasts in hypertrophic scars exhibit a normal response when exposed to growth factors, and show a moderate increase in collagen synthesis.

TGF-β linkage to increased collagen and fibronectin deposition has also been involved in the pathogenesis of excessive scarring. Furthermore, collagen fibers in these types of scars are found to be arranged as whorled, hyalinized bundles. Even though angiogenesis usually regresses during the maturation phase of the normal scarring process, keloids and scars are characterized by persistent hyperemia due to the constant presence of new vessels in the area. Other factors implicated in the development of hypertrophic scars and keloids are hyaluronic acid, proteoglycans, and mast cells, among others.

## Pathogenesis of Atrophic Scars

Atrophic scars are commonly seen in patients with a history of acne; however other conditions such as varicella, surgery, and trauma may also cause atrophic scarring.

Acne lesions usually arise from the pilosebaceous follicles, which initially get obstructed with horny cells. Then a closed or open comedo usually develops, which may later become inflamed. The presence of *Propionibacterium acnes* is essential in the development of inflammatory acne.

The follicular thinning of the wall may result in rupture of the hair follicle with stimulation of a foreign body reaction and activation of the complement cascade. At this point, an attempt to limit the inflammatory reaction by epidermal encapsulation occurs. It is the degree of inflammation that determines the risk and amount of post-acne scarring.

This way acne scarring originates from a deep inflammatory reaction, and involves the destruction or loss of connective tissue, with dermal

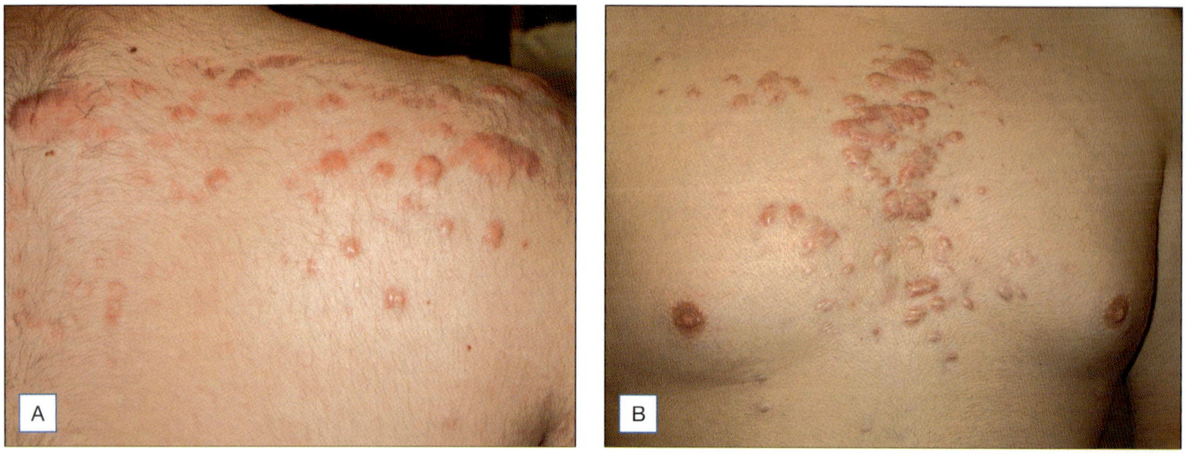


**Fig. 4.4** Keloid-type acne scarring located on the back (**A**) and chest (**B**) of a Caucasian man

atrophy and fibrosis. During the maturation phase, the scar contracts and pulls the surface layers, causing indentation of the skin.

Even though atrophic scars are the most common type of post-acne scarring, some patients may also present with hypertrophic scars and keloids (Fig. 4.4 A and B).

## Expected Benefits

### Pulsed-dye laser

The PDL belongs to the vascular-specific laser group. The PDL, with a wavelength of 585 or 595 nm, was originally created for the treatment of vascular lesions such as hemangiomas and port-wine stains.

The PDL was initially found to be useful in the treatment of scars, when improvement in erythema and skin texture was noted after treating argon-induced scarring. Over the years, many studies have shown significant improvement in scar erythema, texture, height, pliability as well as pruritus, when treating both hypertrophic and keloidal scars. In burn scars, a significant improvement of the intense pruritus, within days of PDL treatment, has also been reported.

Scar improvement after one to two PDL treatment sessions has been reported to be between 57% and 83%.

The mechanism by which the PDL improves the appearance of scars has not been determined. However, theories such as microvascular destruction with consequent ischemia, leading to deprivation of nutrients to the scar and interference in collagen deposition have been proposed. Other hypotheses include the presence of an increased number of mast cells with release of histamine, which affects dermal collagen, disulfide bond disruption, and collagenolysis.

More recently, molecular studies have associated regression of keloids after PDL treatment with the suppression of fibroblast proliferation, upregulation of matrix metalloproteinases-13, induction of apoptosis and mitogen-activated protein kinase activity, and downregulation of TGF-β1, among others.

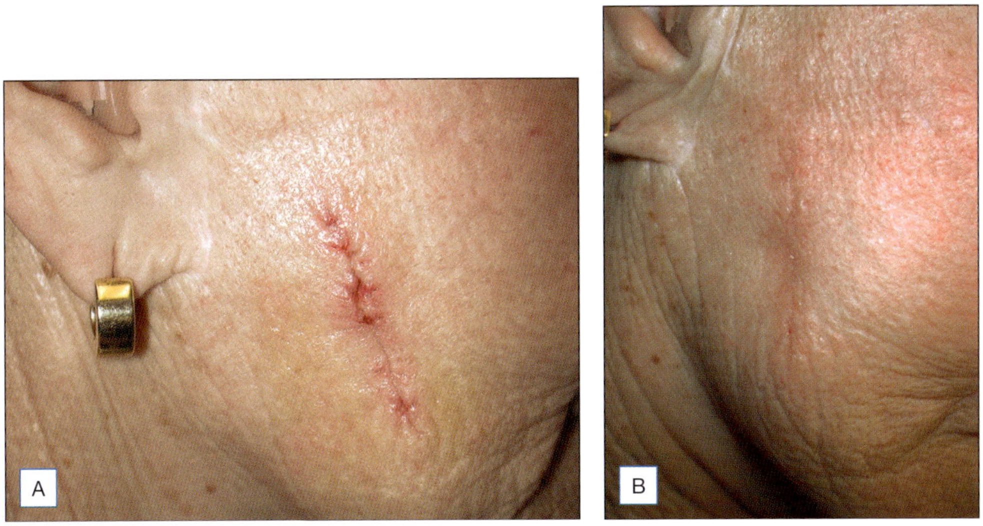


**Fig. 4.5** (**A**) Normal-appearing post-surgical linear scar located on the face of a Caucasian female patient on the day of suture removal. (**B**) Same patient 1 month after PDL treatment over the entire scar

In general, improvement of the scar's erythema, height, and pliability as well as relief of associated symptoms such as pruritus can be expected after treatment with the PDL (Fig. 4.5 A and B).

## Carbon dioxide laser

The carbon dioxide ($CO_2$) laser emits light at a wavelength of 10,600 nm and targets the water-containing tissue. The original $CO_2$ laser was created in a continuous wave (CW) mode, which allowed a constant emission of beam light. This CW mode exposed the tissues to the laser energy for an extended period of time, which resulted in injury of nontargeted tissue with a high incidence of necrosis and scarring. This led to the development of a pulsed mode and scanned $CO_2$ laser device, which delivers high energy in short-duration pulses (less than 1 ms), thus allowing a more controlled ablation of the targeted tissue with fewer complications.

The treating physician is able to control the amount and depth of tissue to be ablated depending on the number of passes performed over the surface to be treated and the energy used. One single pass achieves tissue vaporization depths of 20–60 μm with additional thermal necrosis of 20–50 μm.

Review of the literature by Jordan et al reported improvement ranging form 25–90% of atrophic scarring after $CO_2$ laser resurfacing. Alster and West found an average of 81.4% clinical improvement in 50 patients with moderate to severe acne scarring treated with a high-energy, short-pulsed $CO_2$ laser.

Collagen shrinkage, neocollagenesis and collagen remodeling are believed to be the main factors associated to the long-term clinical improvement seen after $CO_2$ laser resurfacing.

## Er:YAG laser

The short-pulsed erbium:yttrium-aluminum-garnet (Er:YAG) laser has a wavelength of 2940 nm and a pulse duration of 250 μs, and a higher coefficient of absorption than that of the $CO_2$ laser, making the Er:YAG laser 12–18 times more readily absorbed by water-containing tissue. It was developed in an effort to achieve clinical improvement comparable to that with the $CO_2$ laser, but with fewer side effects. This laser penetrates an average of 2–5 μm per J/cm$^2$ with thermal necrosis extending another 10–15 μm. Owing to its limited thermal injury, vascular coagulation is minimal, resulting in poor hemostasis during the procedure. In addition, collagen contraction is also limited and therefore clinical outcome is less significant. On the other hand, the possibility of ablating tissue in a controlled manner and having limited collateral thermal injury results in fewer side effects and faster recovery in comparison to the carbon dioxide laser.

In an effort to overcome the limitations of the short-pulsed Er:YAG laser (e.g. poor hemostasis and superficial tissue ablation) a dual-mode Er:YAG laser (short and long pulsed) was developed. It allows deeper tissue ablation with improved intraoperative hemostasis, as well as increased collagen contraction.

A study by Jeong et al evaluated the effectiveness of the long-pulsed Er:YAG laser in 35 patients with pitted facial acne scars. Through evaluation of photographs, two independent physicians found a clinical improvement average of 71%. In a more recent study by Tanzi and colleagues, treatment of 25 patients with moderate to severe atrophic acne scarring was done using the dual-mode Er:YAG laser. They reported an average score improvement of 2.16 (score scale from 1–3, with a score of 2 meaning 51–75% improvement) 12 months after treatment.

Woo et al recently compared the effectiveness of short-pulsed, variable-pulsed, and dual-mode Er:YAG lasers for the treatment of different types of atrophic acne scarring. They concluded that when treating rolling and deep boxcar scars, the long-pulsed Er:YAG type is more efficient. Whereas, treatment of shallow boxcar and icepick scars may be successfully done with any of the Er:YAG laser types used in the study.

Treatment of facial atrophic acne scars with the Er:YAG laser may achieve an average visual clinical improvement of 50%.

Some laser surgeons currently use both the $CO_2$ and Er:YAG lasers for facial skin resurfacing on the same patient. A total of 24 patients were surveyed 30 months after undergoing facial skin resurfacing with combination $CO_2$/Er:YAG treatment; they were asked about their experience and results of the treatment. A total of 71% of patients indicated that they would undergo the procedure again, and 88% thought their appearance had improved. The patients rated their final appearance on a scale ranging from 0–3 (mean 1.8).

## Nonablative: diode 1450 and Nd:YAG 1320 lasers

Nonablative laser therapy for the treatment of atrophic scars is a relatively new technology. This type of laser treatment targets water-containing tissues without ablating or injuring the epidermis, therefore allowing the patient to resume daily activities immediately after treatment.

There are several laser devices on the market that have been used for nonablative purposes such as the PDL, 1064 nm Q-switched Nd:YAG, Erbium:glass 1540 nm, Nd:YAG 1320 nm, and diode 1450 nm, among others. The 1320 nm Nd:YAG and the diode 1450 nm are currently the two most widely used devices for nonablative treatment of facial atrophic scarring.

The newest version of the 1320 nm Nd:YAG laser has incorporated, in addition to the cryogen spray, a dynamic thermal sensing device that is able to detect the temperature of the epidermis during treatment. If the temperature falls out of an established range (32–34°C), this device is able to halt further firing of the laser to adequately protect the epidermis from thermal damage. Furthermore, this laser system allows cooling immediately before and after laser irradiation.

The 1450 nm diode laser (Smoothbeam, Candela Corp., Wayland, MA) also belongs to the infrared nonablative systems. Similar to the 1320 nm, the diode laser is also equipped with a cryogen spray to provide epidermal cooling.

Some studies on the effectiveness of both of these laser systems in the treatment of atrophic acne scarring have been reported in the literature. Tanzi and colleagues compared the efficacy of the Nd:YAG 1320 nm (CoolTouch 3; CoolTouch Corp., Aurburn, CA) and diode 1450 nm (SmoothBeam; Candela Corp., Wayland, MA) lasers in the treatment of mild to moderate atrophic acne scarring, in a split-face trial. A total of 20 patients received three treatments at monthly intervals of the diode laser (single pass at fluences ranging from 9–14 J/cm$^2$) on one side of the face, and two passes of the Nd:YAG laser at fluences of 12–17 J/cm$^2$ over the contralateral side of the face. Evaluation of digital images by independent dermatologists revealed maximum improvement 6 months after treatment for both lasers. Both patients and physicians in this study found a greater improvement of the side treated with the 1450 nm diode laser.

However, other recently published studies have shown that nonablative laser treatment of atrophic acne scarring with the 1320 nm Nd:YAG laser may have a greater improvement when three passes are done in each treatment session.

Sadick et al treated eight patients with atrophic scarring with the 1320 nm Nd:YAG laser (CoolTouch 3, New Star Lasers, Roseville, CA). A total of six treatments at monthly intervals were carried out. Each treatment consisted of three passes of the laser beam (at fluences ranging from 13–18 J/cm$^2$). Significant clinical improvement was seen 5 months and 1 year after treatment (20–39% and 40–59%, respectively). In a previous similar study by Rogachefsky and colleagues, 12 patients underwent a total of three laser treatments with the 1320 nm Nd:YAG. Each treatment consisted of three passes at fluences ranging from 13–22 J/cm$^2$. Their results showed mild improvement of the scarring, which was statistically significant.

Overall, a 40–45% atrophic scar improvement (which corresponds to mild to moderate improvement) has been reported in the literature after treatment with either the 1320 nm or 1450 nm laser, which is generally seen 4–6 months after treatment.

On a personal communication (KA Arndt), 34 patients who underwent nonablative treatment with the 1320 nm Nd:YAG laser (CoolTouch 2; CoolTouch Corp., Roseville, CA) for acne scarring or photoaging reported a 5.4 and 3.8 degree of improvement (scale 0–10), respectively. The majority of the patients noted improvement between the third and fourth treatment sessions.

Nonablative laser therapy produces thermal injury of the dermis without affecting the epidermis, stimulating dermal fibroblasts, which induce neocollagenesis as well as collagen remodeling. Histologic analysis of biopsy specimens taken from laser-treated areas show new collagen formation 6 months after treatment.

The effectiveness of new nonablative monopolar radiofrequency devices is being studied. A dual effect, with decrease of active acne lesions as well as improvement of acne scarring has been reported by Ruiz-Esparza. These devices are able to generate electric energy with production of heat through resistance in the dermis, while sparing the epidermis. Further studies are underway to determine the mechanism of action, and adequate treatment protocols.

## Fractional Resurfacing

Fractional resurfacing (Fraxel, Reliant Technologies, Palo Alto, CA) is a recent advancement in skin resurfacing. Localized photothermolysis can improve photodamaged skin and induce collagen remodeling. This laser-assisted procedure is able to attain skin rejuvenation with minimal downtime. What makes this technique different from all others is that it only affects a small portion of the skin, while skin adjacent to the treated spots is unaffected. Laser spots can create nearly 2000 microscopic zones 70–100 μm in diameter in 1 $cm^2$; the zones typically are 200–300 μm apart. After fractional resurfacing, the collagen in these microwounds remodels as the sites heal. As only a portion of the skin is injured, patients recover quickly after treatment.

Fractional resurfacing has been used to treat both acne and post-surgical scars. Following several treatments (approximately four to five), these scars demonstrated improved texture, contour, and appearance.

## Plasma Rejuvenation/Resurfacing

Although not a laser, plasma skin resurfacing is a recent advancement in cosmetic dermatology. It utilizes millisecond pulses of nitrogen plasma to induce skin regeneration. By passing radiofrequency pulses into the nitrogen gas, this technology is able to heat the targeted skin. The result is specific tissue ablation with minimal underlying injury. The plasma pulses thermally remodel the underlying skin and create an environment conducive to improvement in many conditions including wrinkles as well as skin texture, contour, and coloration. Plasma resurfacing can utilize multiple low-energy treatments or single high-energy treatments. With this technology, rapid skin heating is achieved while being well tolerated by patients. Side effects may include mild erythema and desquamation. Biopsies have shown full skin regeneration achieved within 1 week after plasma treatment. Currently it is used for facial wrinkles and tightening. In addition, a recent study by Potter et al demonstrated a 35% decrease in acne scar depth after plasma skin resurfacing; notably, no skin coloration changes or scarring was observed after treatment. Such improvements may be seen with other scars, but more studies are warranted to realize the full potential of this new technique.

## Overview of Treatment Strategy

### Treatment approach

#### *Hypertrophic scars and keloids*

As previously explained, the Nd:YAG and $CO_2$ lasers were used in the past for hypertrophic scar revision; however, the elevated recurrence rates and unacceptable side effects, such as pigmentation alteration, led to their decreased use.

Currently, the laser of choice for the treatment of hypertrophic scars and keloids is the PDL. Although established hypertrophic scars can respond to treatment, early treatment of scars within the first months after injury usually results in a better outcome and may also prevent hypertrophy in individuals who are keloid prone. The 585 nm PDL has been shown by Nouri to be safe and effective for treatment in improving the appearance and quality of scars starting on the day of suture removal.

The type of scar that shows the best results and is therefore ideal for PDL treatment is a relatively new scar (less than 1 year old) that is still erythematous or red. Older scars appear less red, and tend to be similar to the surrounding skin color or hypopigmented. These older scars may partially respond to PDL treatment, but it is usually recommended to use some type of adjunctive therapy such as intralesional steroids, 5-FU, or occlusive therapy with silicone gel sheets, among others. Silicone gel sheeting has been used for both prophylaxis and treatment of hypertrophic scars and keloids (Fig. 4.6). Satisfactory results have been reported to occur with regular daily use for 2–4 months.

Studies comparing PDL treatment alone or combined with intralesional corticosteroid have been carried out. Improvements in scars with both treatment protocols were seen without a significant difference between the two approaches. Manuskiatti and Fitzpatrick compared scar treatment with intralesional corticosteroids alone or combined with 5-FU or 5-FU alone or PDL (585 nm, PhotoGenica V; Cynosure Inc., Chelmsford, MA) using fluences of 5 J/cm$^2$ with a 10 mm spot size and 450 μs pulse duration. All treatment areas were improved compared to baseline, however there was no significant difference in treatment outcome compared to method of treatment. They concluded that treatment with intralesional corticosteroids alone

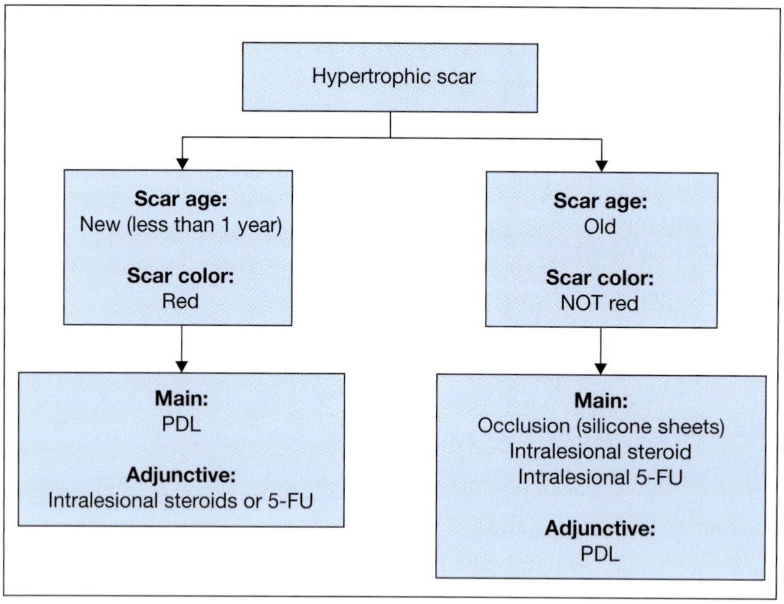


**Fig. 4.6** Treatment approach for hypertrophic scars

or in combination with 5-FU or 5-FU alone and PDL treatment are comparable.

## *Atrophic scars*

There are nonsurgical and surgical treatments for atrophic acne scarring. Nonsurgical procedures include dermal fillers (including bovine collagen, human collagen, hyaluronic acid, and autologous fat, among others), chemical peeling and microdermabrasion. Surgical methods include punch excision, punch elevation, subcision, dermal grafting, and laser surgery (Fig. 4.6).

Currently there are two main laser approaches for atrophic scarring, either ablative resurfacing or nonablative treatment. The procedure, recovery time, and degree of improvement are totally different for both of these laser treatment approaches. The physician must decide which treatment approach is adequate for each particular patient depending on the degree of scarring, the patient's expectations regarding the amount of time needed to achieve noticeable results, and the flexibility of the patient's schedule to allow recovery time.

Many physicians have experienced further improvement of the scars when combination of surgical revision (e.g. punch excision, punch elevation, or subcision) followed by ablative skin resurfacing (e.g. $CO_2$, Er:YAG, or combination $CO_2$/Er:YAG) is carried out.

## *Striae distensae*

Striae distensae, also known as stretch marks, are types of atrophic scars. Initially, they can appear as pink, erythematous areas of thinned skin, which gradually become darker. As the striae mature, they acquire a white coloration parallel to skin tension lines. Unfortunately, no consistent treatment has been found for striae. Topical retinoic acid may improve the skin's appearance.

Since striae are types of scars, it seemed appropriate that lasers could also improve these lesions through collagen remodeling. A 585 nm PDL (Photogenica V; Cynosure, Bedford, MA) is often used with a 450 μs pulse duration. The most advantageous treatment parameters were shown to be 3 J/cm$^2$ with a 10 mm spot size while they are still red or pink; however, fluences from 2–4 J/cm$^2$, with either 7 or 10 mm spot sizes, also led to some improvement. These are nonpurpuric settings and the stretch marks significantly improved in the months following laser treatment. The PDL is not recommended for darker Fitzpatrick skin types IV–VI, because there is a significant risk of skin dyspigmentation, purpura, and postinflammatory hyperpigmentation. $CO_2$ and Er:YAG lasers have also been tried, but are not recommended for removing striae.

Infrared lasers are another option that may show gradual improvement with multiple treatments or in combination with other modalities. These lasers are safe in those with sun-tanned skin and darker skin types. Intense pulsed light (broad spectrum 515–1200 nm) has been shown to significantly improve striae. Patients in one study underwent five sessions, and all patients saw at least some improvement in their stretch marks, with 60% demonstrating good to very good improvement. These results are promising since the treated lesions were all white, older striae that are usually more difficult to treat.

Finally, at least one study has shown that fractional photothermolysis, with its ablative and nonablative properties, can be an effective method for improving the contour, texture, and appearance of mature stretch marks. More studies are needed, but this and other new modalities, such as plasma rejuvenation/resurfacing, may prove to be safe and effective treatments. Currently, there is no single effective treatment that is able to remove striae in all people. Striae are difficult to treat and typically require multiple treatments to demonstrate any improvement. Patients should have realistic expectations. Treatments may improve striae, but will not likely remove them completely. Newer, pink striae may be more appropriately treated with a PDL. Older, white striae may respond to numerous treatments with intense pulsed light.

## Major determinants

### *Skin type*

The skin type of the patient is not only the initial patient feature that is noticed by the physician, but it is also a main factor to be taken into account when considering scar revision with lasers. As it was previously explained, treatment of hypertrophic scars with the PDL may be done in dark-skinned individuals; however, a higher risk of pigmentation alteration is present. Some physicians do not recommend PDL treatment in patients with skin types IV–VI. In an effort to decrease pigmentation side effects, those physicians who do treat these patients with hypertrophic scars and keloids with PDL suggest decreasing the energy settings. When the fluence is decreased, more treatment sessions might be needed to achieve the desired scar improvement. In addition, doing a 'test spot' is also recommended in an effort to foresee any undesired side effects and to better determine initial laser parameters to be used.

Both the 585 PDL and 532 nm Q-switched Nd:YAG laser have been shown to be effective in the treatment of pigmented hypertrophic scars, with 38% and 36% improvement, respectively. In addition, the 532 nm Q-switched Nd:YAG laser had a more significant effect on the scar color, while the 585 nm PDL had a more pronounced effect on the scar's pliability and height. The PDL, however, remains the laser of choice for the treatment of hypertrophic scars and keloids.

In the case of ablative skin resurfacing with the $CO_2$ or Er:YAG laser, there is a risk of pigmentation alteration for all patients no matter the skin type; however, once again there is a higher risk of post-inflammatory hyperpigmentation in darker skinned individuals, which is usually temporary. The Er:YAG laser may be somewhat preferred over the carbon dioxide laser when treating patients with skin types IV–VI, due to its shorter recovery period and less hyperpigmentation. Non-ablative laser therapy is associated with a lower risk of postinflammatory hyperpigmentation; however, it may still occur in dark-skinned individuals. Compared to that of resurfacing techniques, postinflammatory hyperpigmentation occurring after nonablative therapy usually appears to be less severe and resolves faster.

### *Age of the scar*

This is another major determinant when considering PDL treatment. As previously explained, scars that are less than 1 year old and are still red in color show a better and faster response to laser therapy. For older scars, nonlaser treatments might be considered such as intralesional steroids, 5-FU, as well as occlusive therapy with silicone gel sheets.

### *Type of lesion, extent and severity of acne scarring*

These are other major determinants when deciding which laser to use for a particular patient. When only a few atrophic scars are present, spot resurfacing may be considered, preceded or not by punch excision, punch elevation, or subcision. However, when numerous lesions need to be addressed, then ablative resurfacing or nonablative treatment of the entire cosmetic unit must be undertaken in order to achieve a more uniform or even outcome.

Several sessions (four to six) of nonablative laser treatment are usually required to achieve mild to moderate improvement of the lesions. Comparison on the degree of improvement achieved by ablative and nonablative therapies is a controversial issue. Many physicians believe that the degree of improvement of nonablative treatment is comparable to that of full-face resurfacing. Therefore, laser skin resurfacing is currently being performed less frequently than nonablative therapy for the treatment of atrophic scarring.

On the other hand, other laser surgeons believe that evidence on the clinical outcome achieved by the nonablative approach is mild and not as remarkable as ablative techniques.

### *Recovery time*

Recovery time is not an issue when treating hypertrophic scars or keloids with the PDL. However, when facial resurfacing via the $CO_2$ or Er:YAG lasers is chosen for the treatment of acne scarring, downtime is definitely another main factor to be discussed with the patient. Patients undergoing ablative skin resurfacing usually require 7–12 days of recovery time, until complete re-epithelialization occurs. If the patient desires a less invasive treatment that allows them to go back to their life activities immediately, newer nonablative therapies are the current alternatives. However, initial noticeable results with the nonablative lasers are usually seen approximately 4–6 months (in three to five treatment sessions) after the last treatment session.

### *Cost and number of treatments*

Cost and number of treatments should be discussed with patients when deciding treatment options for scar revision. Laser scar revision is usually considered a cosmetic treatment, thus the majority of insurance companies do not cover these expenses. In the case of PDL for hypertrophic scars and keloids, as well as nonablative treatment for acne scarring, multiple sessions (approximately three or four) are required at monthly intervals to achieve the desired effect. On the other hand, ablative resurfacing of the skin is usually done in one treatment session; however, it is a longer and more invasive surgical procedure that involves not only the use of anesthesia, but also more personnel and recovery time that limits (in the majority of cases) the return of the patient to work for at least 1 week. All of these factors determine a higher cost per session compared to nonablative therapy and PDL. However, at the end, depending on each physician's practice fees, the total cost for four to six nonablative treatment sessions may still be less than a full-face laser resurfacing.

### *Patient interviews*

Patients' expectations, cosmetic and symptomatic, need to be addressed prior to starting any treatment. It is crucial for the physician to explain that total eradication of the scars should not be expected.

Inflammatory conditions (such as acne or varicella) as well as infections (e.g. herpes zoster) must be under control or resolved before undergoing laser treatment of the resulting scars. Laser treatment that is performed during an inflammatory process or infection may result in dissemination of the infection, increased inflammation followed by further scarring, and higher risk of other side effects.

Determining the history of the scar or keloid in terms of: age, evolution, and previous treatments is important; as previously stated, the sooner the scar is treated, the better results will be achieved. Newly formed scars that are only red may not need further treatment due to the likelihood of clearance with time, as the scar matures. However, newly formed scars that are red and start becoming hypertrophic with time, or in those patients who are keloid prone, may greatly be improved with early laser treatment. Patients may present with a history of previously failed attempts to improve the appearance of their scars. Previous treatments with other nonlaser modalities may cause increased fibrosis of the scar, resulting in a lesion that is more difficult to treat.

The skin type of the patient must be determined according to the Fitzpatrick classification. The majority of patients suffering from hypertrophic scars and keloids have Fitzpatrick skin types IV–VI. As explained before, although these patients may benefit from laser treatment of their hypertrophic scars, there is a high risk of pigmentation alteration as a side effect. It is of high importance for the treating physician to notify the patient of the high probability of hyperpigmentation. Nevertheless, it is likely that the patient will decide to continue with the procedure regardless of this risk. These patients usually consider that the cosmetic burden caused by their pathologic scars is much greater than the resulting hyperpigmentation.

Patients with acne must be questioned about the previous or current use of isotretinoin. Suspension of the medication for at least 6–12 months is recommended before performing any scar revision procedure, due to a higher risk of developing hypertrophic scars.

## Treatment Techniques

### Pulsed-dye laser

PDL treatment of hypertrophic scars and keloids is an outpatient procedure which is usually well tolerated without use of anesthetic. If the patient requests it, a topical anesthetic can be placed on the scar 30–60 minutes before the laser treatment. Any residual anesthetic, as well as any make-up, must be removed with soap and water before the procedure to prevent it from interfering with light absorption.

Previous to the laser treatment, evaluation of the scar in terms of size, color, height, and associated symptoms must be carried out at every visit and by the same person. Also, pictures of the lesion before each session should be taken to follow progressive improvement of the scar. It is always recommended to use the same camera, lighting and distance, in order to maintain a standardized image.

Every person present in the room for the procedure must wear appropriate eye protection according to the lasers' wavelength. Inform the patient that you are about to start the procedure, and explain that he or she will experience a 'rubber band snapping' discomfort during the treatment.

The laser must be calibrated and parameters to be used must be set according to the manufacturer's instructions for the laser to be used.

In general, the following are the parameters that are most commonly used at the current authors' clinic (PhotoGenica VLS; Cynosure Inc., Chelmsford, MA): wavelength 585 nm, pulse duration 450 μs, spot size 10 mm, and fluences ranging from 3–4 J/mm$^2$. When using smaller handpieces (5 or 7 mm) the energy settings must be increased. Initial treatment visits should be started with low fluences, which can be adjusted according to the response in subsequent sessions. When starting on suture removal day, in a clinical study by Nouri et al, the 585 nm PDL (Cynosure Inc., Chelmsford, MA) was used at monthly intervals (total three treatments) with a 10 mm spot size at 3.5 J/cm$^2$. These particular settings were nonpurpura inducing. In her original studies involving hypertrophic scars, Dr Alster used 585 nm PDL (Candela Laser Corp., Wayland, MA) with a 450 μs and fluence between 6.5 and 6.75 J/cm$^2$; no spot size was specified. In another study, Alster et al treated sternotomy scars with the same laser and wavelength, but with a 5 mm spot size and a mean fluence of 7.0 J/cm$^2$. For burn scars, they used the PDL with a pulse duration of 450–1500 μs, 4.5–5.0 J/cm$^2$ (10 mm spot) and 5.0–6.5 J/cm$^2$ (7 mm spot). These parameters are likely to be purpuric. A comparison on the effectiveness between shorter (e.g. 450 μs) and longer (e.g. 1.5 ms) pulse durations for the treatment of hypertrophic scars, to the current authors' knowledge, has not been reported. However, it is their assumption that long pulse durations would be less effective.

Proceed by placing the handpiece over one end of the scar and start applying laser pulses over the entire scar surface in a continuous pattern until reaching the opposite end (Fig. 4.7 A–C). Overlapping of 10% is generally accepted.

**Postoperative care instructions** should include strict sun avoidance to prevent pigmentation alterations. The treated area may be normally cleansed with soap and water, and make-up is not contraindicated. The next treatment session should be arranged in 4–6 weeks (Fig. 4.8 A–C).

**Expected side effects** include a burning or pruritic sensation that is usually noticed immediately after the procedure and may persist from a few hours up to 2 days.

The current authors usually recommend using nonpurpuric induction parameters when treating scars. However, if purpura does develop, it is limited to the treated area and may last between 7–10 days (Fig. 4.7B). The affected area may be covered with make-up immediately after the treatment session.

Transient hyperpigmentation may also occur. In such cases, the following treatment session must be deferred until resolution to avoid light absorption by epidermal melanin and assure appropriate targeting. Bleaching creams may also be indicated for faster resolution.

**Complications** such as crusting, oozing and vesiculation are rare, but sometimes occur. In such cases, the area should be kept moist with ointment (e.g. petrolatum jelly) and may be covered with a nonstick occlusive dressing to avoid touching of the area. Complete healing of the site must be achieved before the following treatment session, time at which lower energy settings should be used.

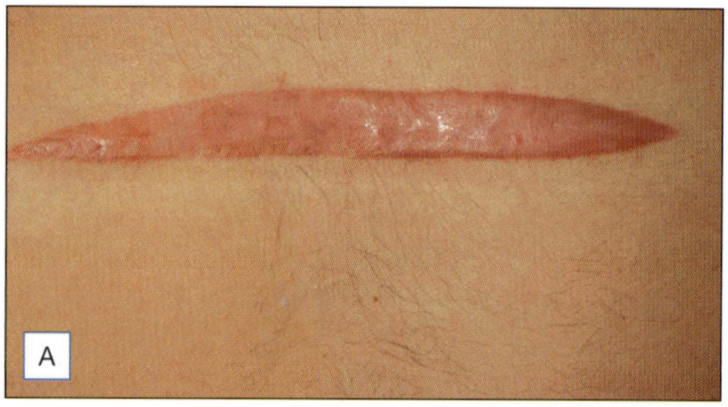


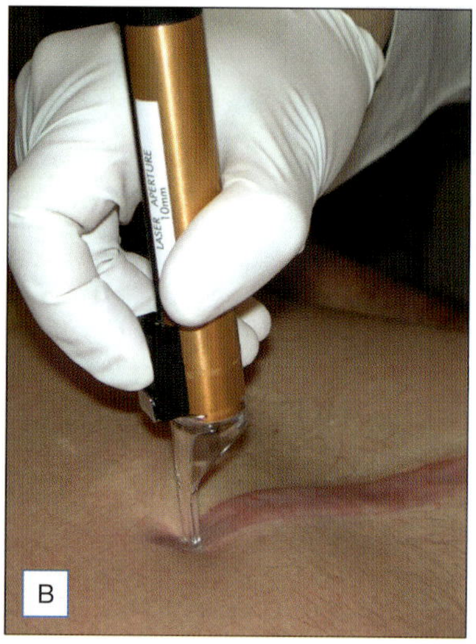


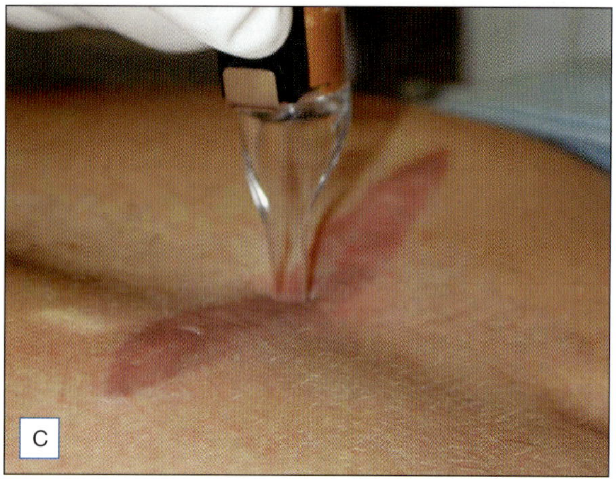


**Fig. 4.7** (**A**) Hypertrophic linear scar located on the chest of a male patient. Start laser treatment by placing the handpiece in one end of the scar (**B**) and apply pulses over the entire scar surface in a continuous pattern (**C**)

## Laser resurfacing

Laser skin resurfacing is an invasive procedure that requires administration of anesthetics. Depending on the surface area to be treated, either nerve block or conscious sedation by an anesthesiologist is indicated.

Once again all make-up must be removed prior to treatment. The degree and type of scarring must be recorded, however it is more important to obtain pre-treatment pictures of the affected area. New images in follow-up visits should be taken using the same camera, lighting and distance, in order to maintain a standardized image and compare the clinical outcome.

Every person present in the room for the procedure must wear eye protection as well as masks that cover the mouth and nose. Tissue ablation during the procedure may produce vaporization of particles that may be hazardous, and therefore protection of the airways must be undertaken. In addition, vacuum devices should be used during the procedure to absorb and filter the smoke. The eyes of the patient should be protected with saline-soaked gauze.

The laser parameters should be set according to the manufacturer's instructions. After each laser pass, partially desiccated tissue accumulates on the surface. This tissue must be completely removed with saline-soaked gauze to prevent further thermal necrosis of the tissue.

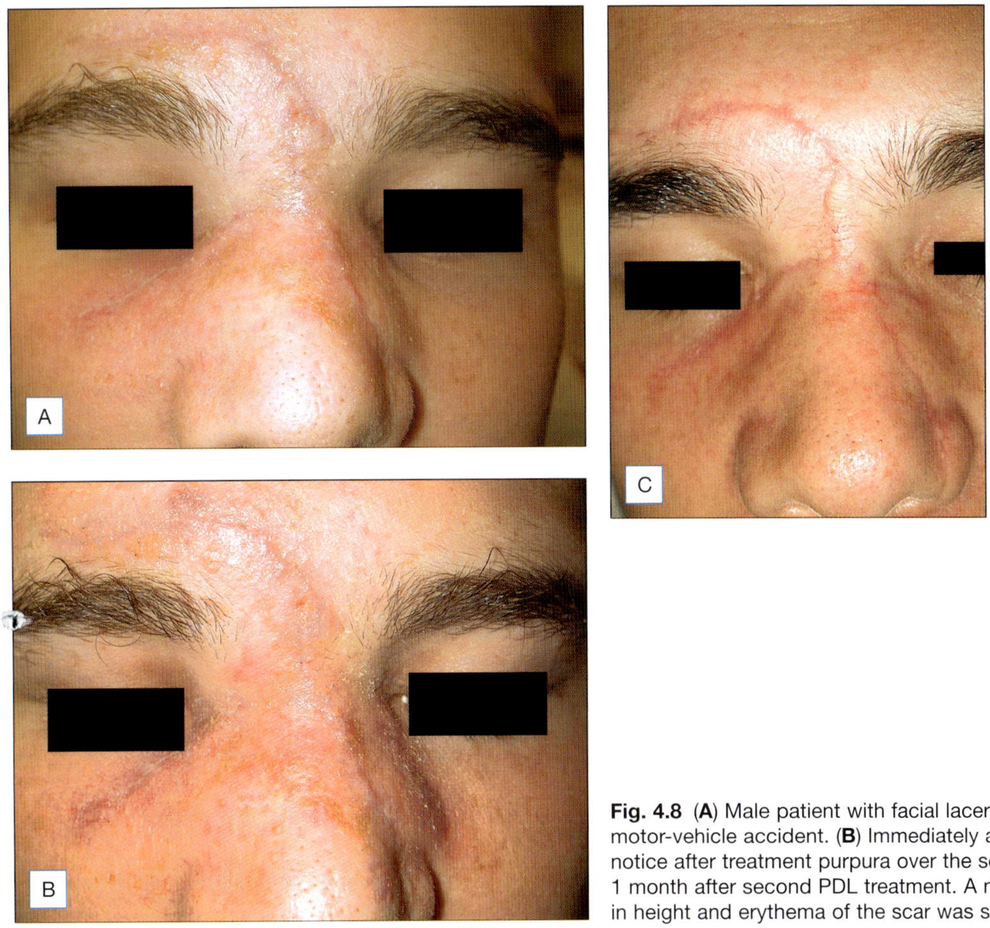


**Fig. 4.8** (**A**) Male patient with facial lacerations 3 weeks after motor-vehicle accident. (**B**) Immediately after PDL treatment: notice after treatment purpura over the scar. (**C**) Same patient 1 month after second PDL treatment. A noticeable decrease in height and erythema of the scar was seen

Multiple passes (one to three) are usually required for treatment of atrophic scars with both the $CO_2$ and Er:YAG lasers. However, the physician must remember that the purpose of this treatment method is to reduce the depth of the scar and stimulate collagen remodeling, which will later level the remaining defect.

**Postoperative care includes** either the closed or open methods. The current authors' method includes the placement of a semiocclusive dressing or net stocking (e.g. Flexzan, Vigilon) over the lasered area, which is left in place for 48–72 hours. Placement of cold compresses is also recommended to reduce the swelling. Once the dressing is removed, the patient is asked to frequently apply a thick ointment such as petrolatum jelly (i.e. Vaseline) over the entire treatment site. Some physicians prefer no to use the semiocclusive dressing technique, allowing the patient to start applying cold compresses and healing ointment as soon as possible (open); whereas others maintain the semi-occlusive method during the entire re-epithelialization period.

Laser resurfacing may cause activation of latent herpes simplex virus (HSV) infection or can induce a primary HSV infection of the patient during the recovery period. Therefore, antiviral prophylaxis starting

48 hours before or the same day of laser surgery is usually accepted as part of the resurfacing protocol, and is usually maintained throughout the re-epithelialization period (e.g. typically only one of these anti-viral agents would be used at a time; acyclovir, famvir, or valtrex).

As has been mentioned before, the recovery time for patients treated with the Er:YAG laser is shorter than for those treated with the $CO_2$ laser.

Expected side effects immediately after treatment include swelling, erythema, and serous discharge or oozing. These side effects gradually and spontaneously decrease with time as re-epithelialization occurs. The intensity of the erythema is proportional to the number of laser passes performed. It usually persists from 1–6 months for patients treated with the $CO_2$ laser, whereas a study by Alster showed that those treated with the Er:YAG laser may experience erythema for a few weeks after the procedure.

Other side effects include acne, milia, contact dermatitis (more common when the patient uses topical antibiotics or ointments containing fragrances), infection (bacterial, viral, and fungal), hyperpigmentation, hypopigmentation, ectropion, and hypertrophic scarring.

Postinflammatory hyperpigmentation is a very common side effect, and usually occurs 3–4 weeks after laser resurfacing. Patients with any skin tone may be affected; however, dark-skinned individuals are typically involved. The hyperpigmentation usually resolves spontaneously within a few months; however, topical bleaching creams may be indicated to accelerate its resolution.

## Nonablative laser

Nonablative treatment of atrophic scarring is a less invasive procedure that is usually well tolerated by patients and may sometimes require the use of topical anesthetics that should be applied to the area to be treated 30–60 minutes before the procedure.

Once again all make-up and any residual anesthetic creams should be completely removed. Baseline pictures should be taken in a standardized manner, so comparison of results may be done after several treatments.

The patient as well as all personnel present in the room during the procedure should wear appropriate eye protection according to the laser's wavelength.

The laser, energy and cooling spray, should be calibrated according to the manufacturer's parameters. Each physician has his or her own technique. In the current authors' clinic, they usually follow a pattern, covering one cosmetic unit at a time, until the entire area to be treated is covered.

A total of four to six treatment sessions at monthly intervals are usually suggested, and results may be expected between 3–6 months after the last laser treatment.

The main advantage of this treatment method is the ability to return to daily activities without any recovery time. Sun avoidance is the main postoperative indication.

Expected side effects immediately after the procedure include erythema that usually disappears within 24 hours.

Rare complications include blistering, crusting, and hyperpigmentation. If blistering or crusting occurs, the patient should be instructed not to touch the area and to keep the lesions moistened with ointment. In addition, postponing the next laser treatment until these lesions resolve should be considered.

## Advanced Topics: Treatment Tips for Experienced Practitioners

When using intralesional corticosteroids or 5-FU in combination with PDL, certain considerations should be taken into account. If using intralesional steroids, it should be done following the laser procedure. The steroids should not be injected into the scar before the laser treatment because it blanches the area, resulting in the risk of losing the laser target (vessel). An average of 10–40 mg/cc immediately can be used after the laser procedure. The current authors routinely use PDL plus intralesional steroids when treating patients with hypertrophic scars or keloids, unless palpation reveals a rather soft and pliable scar tissue.

Many physicians prefer surgical excision of keloids. This is usually done with the least trauma and desiccation possible. However, there is always a high risk of recurrence. Berman et al reported that application of topical imiquimod starting on the same day of surgery may be effective in reducing the risk of recurrence.

### Further Reading

Alster TS 2003 Laser scar revision: Comparison study of 585nm pulsed dye laser with and without intralesional corticosteroids. Dermatologic Surgery 29:25–29

Alster TS, Kurban AK, Grove GL, et al 1993 Alteration of argon laser-induced scars by the pulsed dye laser. Lasers in Surgery and Medicine 13:368–373

Alster TS, West TB 1996 Resurfacing of atrophic facial acne scars with a high-energy, pulsed carbon dioxide laser. Dermatologic Surgery 22:151–155

Berman B, Kaufman J 2002 Pilot study of the effect of postoperative imiquimod 5% cream on the recurrence rate of excised keloids. Journal of the American Academy of Dermatology 47(4 Suppl):S209–S211

Goodman GJ 2000 Management of post-acne scarring: What are the options for treatment? American Journal of Clinical Dermatology 1:3–17

Jeong JT, Kye YC 2001 Resurfacing of pitted facial acne scars with long-pulsed Er:YAG laser. Dermatologic Surgery 27:107–110

Jordan R, Cummins C, Burls A 2000 Laser resurfacing of the skin for the improvement of facial acne scarring: a systematic review of the evidence. Br J Dermatol 142:413–423

Kye YC 1997 Resurfacing of pitted facial scars with a pulsed Er:YAG laser. Dermatologic Surgery 23:880–883

Manuskiatti W, Fitzpatrick RE 2002 Treatment response of keloidal and hypertrophic sternotomy scars: comparison among intralesional corticosteroid, 5-fluorouracil, and 585-nm flashlamp-pumped pulsed-dye laser treatment. Archives of Dermatology 138:1149–1155

Nouri K, Jimenez GP, Harrison-Balestra C, et al 2003 585nm Pulsed dye laser in the treatment of surgical scars starting on the suture removal day. Dermatologic Surgery 29:65–73

Ruiz-Esparza J, Gomez JB 2003 Nonablative radiofrequency for active acne vulgaris: The use of deep dermal heat in the treatment of moderate to severe active acne vulgaris (thermotherapy): a report of 22 patients. Dermatologic Surgery 29:333–339

Sadick NS, Schecter AK 2004 A preliminary study of utilization of the 1320nm Nd:YAG laser for the treatment of acne scarring. Dermatologic Surgery 30:995–1000

Tanzi EL, Alster TS 2002 Treatment of atrophic facial acne scars with a dual-mode Er:YAG laser. Dermatologic Surgery 2002;28:551–555

Tanzi EL, Alster TS 2004 Comparison of a 1450nm diode laser and 1320nm Nd:YAG laser in the treatment of atrophic facial scars: A prospective clinical and histological study. Dermatologic Surgery 30:152–157

Woo SH, Park JH, Kye YC 2004 Resurfacing of different types of facial acne scars with short-pulsed, variable-pulsed, and dual-mode Er:YAG. Dermatologic Surgery 30:448–493

# 5 Effect of Radiation on Wound Healing and Treatment of Scarring

*Roy H. Decker, Lynn D. Wilson*

## Introduction

The clinical effects of ionizing radiation treatment on a cutaneous wound are highly dependent upon the timing of radiation in relation to the process of wound healing, as radiation affects several targets in the processes of inflammation, proliferation, and remodeling. These targets make ionizing radiation one of the most effective treatments for the prophylaxis of hypertrophic scars and keloids. For lesions that have recurred despite more conservative measures, external beam irradiation using either electron beam or kilovoltage range x-rays may be delivered following local excision. Recurrence rates may be decreased following postoperative irradiation. Because the radiation dose used to prevent hyperplasia is significantly lower than that used in the treatment of neoplastic processes, and the dose is delivered superficially with relative sparing of deeper critical structures, the expected acute and chronic morbidity rate of treatment is similarly lower.

## Radiation Treatment Modalities and Definitions

There are several modalities by which external beam radiation therapy can deliver dose to tissue. The selection is made on the basis of depth of the target, nature of critical surrounding structures, and availability. Relevant treatments will be discussed here, for the purpose of understanding the appropriateness of a given radiation prescription.

A photon is a quanta of electromagnetic energy. High-energy photons, in the form of x-rays, are produced by a linear accelerator and are available in a spectrum of energies. They interact with matter primarily via atomic electrons in the target, causing the secondary ionization events by which they deposit their energy. Incident radiation deposits its dose as it passes through matter, becoming attenuated as a function of distance and the properties of the target. Higher energy beams deliver an increased dose at depth in tissue, and relatively less at the surface. Lower energy radiation deposits the dose primarily at the target surface, sparing the deeper matter. Therapeutic photon beams are comprised of a spectrum of frequencies, and practically are specified by their maximum photon energy. The most commonly available treatment energies are in the megavoltage range, which deposit their dose at a range practical for the treatment of targets in human tissue. Such beams were designed to relatively spare surface structures such as skin, which would otherwise be dose limiting, in the interest of delivering a higher dose to deeper target structures. This is in contrast to the more superficial radiation techniques discussed later.

Orthovoltage x-rays refer to photons with maximum energy in the range of 125–400 kV, produced by a dedicated treatment unit. These units are not present in all radiation treatment centers. When available, orthovoltage is often used in dermatologic applications, as the skin surface dose is maximized, and the dose is attenuated rapidly as the beam penetrates deeper into soft tissue.

Grenz rays are even lower energy x-rays in the range of 5–15 kV which were historically used to treat superficial benign epidermal conditions. In these cases, the majority of the target processes are occurring within 1 mm of the skin surface. The majority of grenz-ray radiation is deposited at such shallow depths, and deeper structures such as hair follicles, and sebaceous and sweat glands are relatively spared. Very few grenz-ray machines are still in use in the United States.

Electrons are the product of the same linear accelerators used to produce megavoltage energy photons, and thus are more commonly available than orthovoltage treatment units. Electron beams are commonly used in dermatologic applications as they are capable of delivering a high skin dose, and the deposited dose rapidly falls to negligible values at depth in tissue. Electron depth dose, like that of photons, is a function of voltage. Higher energy electrons deliver dose to a greater depth, similar to the depth/dose relationship of photon energy. Unlike the skin-sparing properties of higher energy photons, however, increasing the energy of electron beams increases the skin dose. Figure 5.1 illustrates the dose deposited by various radiation treatment beams, including electrons, orthovoltage and megavoltage photons, and grenz-rays, as a function of depth in tissue. Such depth dose curves can be manipulated to optimize dose-to-target vs. dose-to-normal structure. For example, **bolus** is a tissue equivalent material that can be placed on the skin surface. The thickness of the bolus can be used to bring the skin dose to a therapeutic level, to spare deeper critical structures, or to provide a flatter treatment surface over highly contoured anatomy to ensure homogenous dose distribution (Figs 5.2–5.5).

In contrast to the external beam modalities discussed earlier, brachytherapy refers to the application of radioactive sources in close proximity to the target. Brachytherapy can be delivered via a permanent implant, such as the placement of radioactive iodine seeds that decay to background over months and remain, inert, in the target tissue thereafter. Alternatively, high-dose rate brachytherapy can be delivered by the placement of catheters in target tissue into which, for example, a radioactive iridium source is briefly placed. This latter treatment is usually repeated a number of times, after which the catheters or other

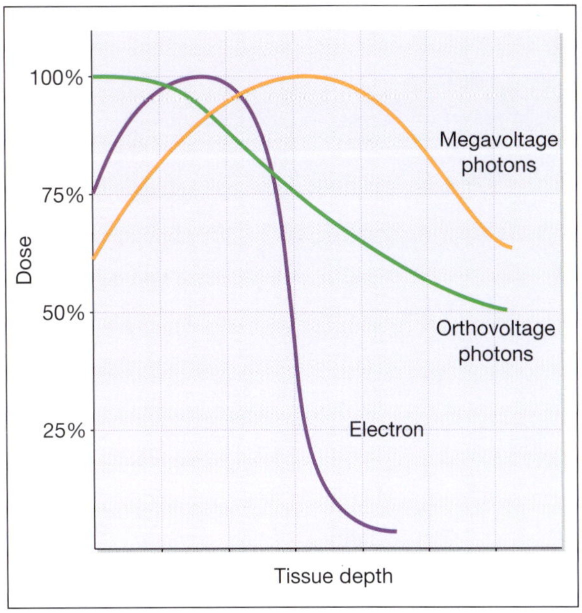


**Fig. 5.1** Depth dose curves of various radiation treatment modalities. Therapeutic ionizing radiation deposits energy in tissue as a function of depth. Photon beams deliver their dose at depth in tissue, and are relatively skin sparing. Orthovoltage x-rays deliver maximum dose to the skin surface, while further dose deposition is rapidly attenuated

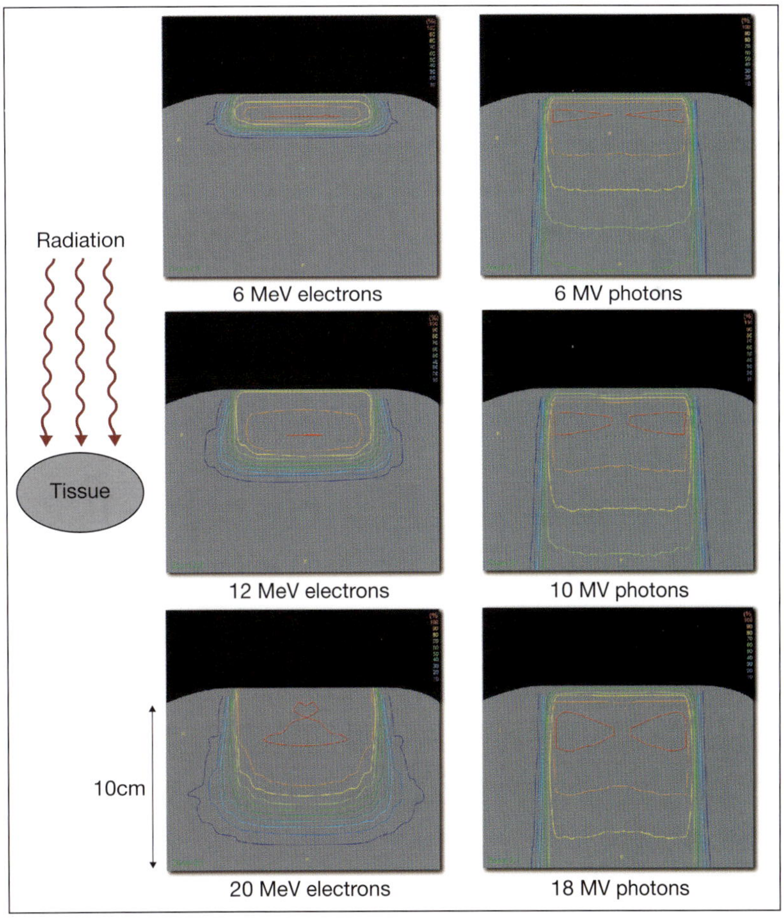


**Fig. 5.2** Dose distribution in tissue varies with energy. Representations of dose distribution in tissue for increasing electron energy (left column) and photon energy (right column). A single radiation beam incident upon the superior aspect of a tissue-equivalent material (grey) will deposit its dose as a function of depth. The lines represent contours of equal dose deposition. For photon energies, after a build-up at shallow depths, dose falls off gradually with depth. For electron energies, this fall-off is more rapid. The total depth shown in each figure is approximately 10 cm

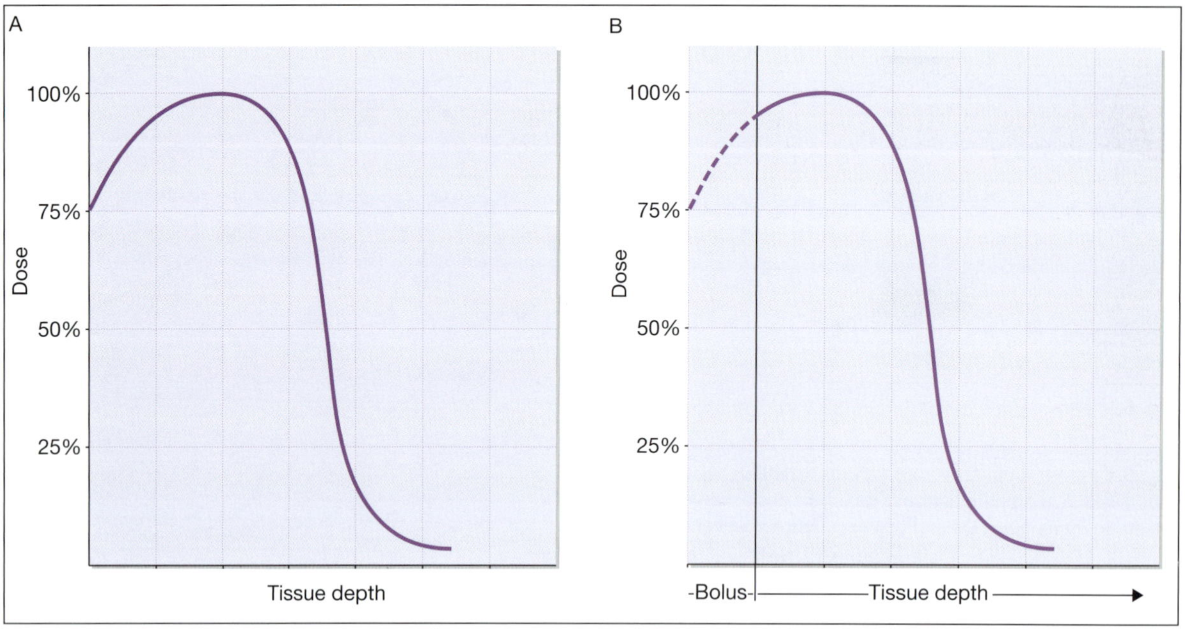


**Fig. 5.3** The use of bolus to alter the depth dose properties of electron beams. (**A**) demonstrates the depth dose properties of electron beams. Dose deposition rises rapidly, then falls to negligible values. (**B**) shows how tissue-equivalent bolus material is used to raise the skin surface dose to maximum, while sparing tissue at depth

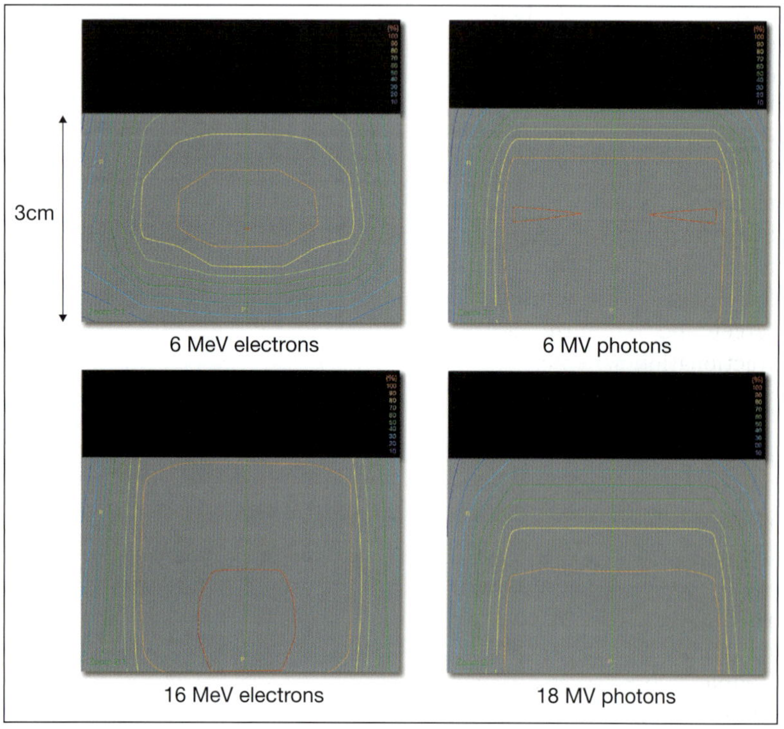


**Fig. 5.4** The skin-sparing properties of high-energy photons. A comparison of the superficial dose deposition of electron beam (left column) vs. photon beam (right column) radiation. The beam is incident downwards upon the superior aspect of a tissue equivalent material (grey). The depth of tissue shown is approximately 3 cm. For electron beams, increasing the beam energy increases surface dose as well as dose at depth. For photon beams, increasing the beam energy decreases surface dose while it increases dose at depth

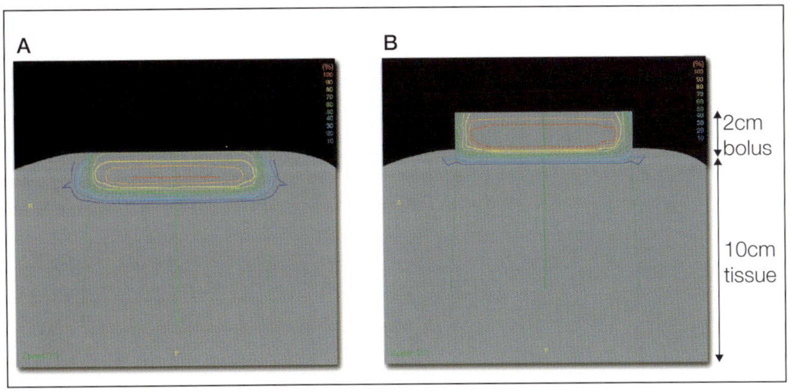


**Fig. 5.5** The use of bolus to increase surface dose and decrease depth dose. The dose distribution of 6 MeV electrons on tissue equivalent material (**A**). The dose to superficial tissue is significantly less than 100%, and there is substantial dose deposited several centimeters deep. With the use of bolus (**B**), the superficial tissue dose is 100%, while deeper tissue is spared

application devices may be removed. Another typical application of brachytherapy to treatment of benign and malignant skin targets is the engineering of superficial radioactive plaque sources, which are placed directly on the skin surface.

The SI (Systeme International d'Unites) unit of radiation dose is the gray (Gy), which is defined as a joule of energy absorbed per kilogram of tissue. An alternate unit of absorbed dose, largely replaced by the gray, is the rad (an acronym for radiation absorbed dose). One gray is equal to 100 rad. Dose is specified to the target volume as defined by the treating radiation therapist. Epithelial malignancies, for example, are treated to a total dose in the range of 50–70 Gy, while hypertrophic scars and keloids are commonly prescribed doses in the range of 4–20 Gy.

Fractionation refers to the delivery of specified radiation dose in temporally separate treatments, and is recommended to both increase the efficacy of effects on target tissue and to allow normal irradiated tissue to repair radiation damage. Thus, the schedule of radiation fractionation can be used to both increase efficacy of the dose to the target and minimize radiation damage to normal tissue. Common fractionation schemes using conventional radiotherapy deliver treatments at intervals ranging from twice daily to once per week.

The clinical effect of radiotherapy on human tissue is mediated by the induction of DNA damage and subsequent mitotic cell death. The process begins when incident photons deposit their energy in tissue by ejecting local orbital electrons. These secondary electrons subsequently initiate local ionization events, primarily by reacting with water, although there is some direct action on cellular DNA. Therapeutic electrons, in contrast to photons, are directly ionizing. The oxidized free radical species produced by ionization induce single or double DNA strand breaks, DNA base alterations or loss, and DNA–DNA and DNA–protein cross-links. The inability of the cell to successfully segregate such damaged chromosomes during mitosis will lead to cell death, unless the cell is able to repair the damage.

The rationale of fractionated radiotherapy lies in the **four Rs** of radiation treatment: redistribution, repopulation, reoxygenation, and repair. Because there is a cell cycle dependence of cellular sensitivity to radiotherapy, temporally separate treatments allow the tumor cell population to redistribute after the sensitive population has been depleted. During the interval between treatments the cell cycle distribution returns to its baseline, ensuring that a susceptible target cell population will be present prior to the subsequent fraction. Reoxygenation refers to the dependency on oxygen of the oxidization events induced by radiation. There is significant heterogeneity of oxygenation status within a tumor cell population, and the more highly oxygenated cells are selectively killed. Fractionated treatment allows diffusion of oxygen to relatively hypoxic cells, again ensuring a susceptible target population. Differences in the rapidity of DNA repair processes in normal and neoplastic cells accounts for part of the selectivity of therapeutic radiation for the tumor tissue. The majority of radiation-induced DNA damage is repaired prior to mitosis in all cell types, but because repair in normal tissue is more efficient, subsequent radiation treatment allows for additive DNA damage to be induced selectively in sublethally damaged tumor cells. Repopulation of both normal tissue and tumor cells occurs during a radiation treatment course. The acute side effects of radiotherapy are due to the depletion of normal tissue stem cells, and the repopulation of these is essential to the recovery of normal tissue.

## Effect of Radiation Treatment on Normal Skin

In discussion of the side effects of radiation treatment, it is convenient to separate acute toxicities, those that occur during or shortly after treatment, from late toxicities – those that occur 90 days or more after treatment is completed. Early effects of irradiation are generally due to the depletion of normal tissue stem cells, which must be repopulated after treatment is complete. Late effects, in contrast, may occur after a delay of months or years after treatment, and are due to both parenchymal cell loss and progressive microvascular damage. The appearance and severity of both acute and late effects are a function of the specific tissue tolerances, total dose delivered, and fractionation schedule. For the majority of such effects there are threshold doses, below which no significant risk of side effects is expected, and above which toxicity occurs in a generally dose-dependent manner (Table 5.1). The incidence and severity of late effects is particularly sensitive to individual fraction size, which is the rationale for extended fractionation regimens in high-dose radiation therapy. There are also, however, stochastic effects of irradiation, primarily the risk of inducing second malignancy. In this case it is not felt that there is an absolute threshold dose for such effects, nor a relationship between severity and dose. Instead, the risk of such effects is related to dose in a nonlinear fashion.

| Tissue Sensitivity and Late Effects of Radiotherapy | | |
|---|---|---|
| **Organ** | **Threshold dose*** | **Late effect** |
| Salivary gland | 30 Gy | Xerostomia |
| Lacrimal gland | 30 Gy | Dry eyes |
| Thyroid | 45 Gy | Hypothyroidism |
| Ovaries | 2–3 Gy | Sterilization |
| Testes | 1–2 Gy | Sterilization |
| Breast, adult | 50 Gy | Atrophy, necrosis |
| Breast, child | 10 Gy | Hypoplasia |
| Eye, retina | 45 Gy | Blindness |
| Eye, lens | 6–10 Gy | Cataracts |
| Lymphatics | 50 Gy | Sclerosis |
| Cartilage/bone, child | 10 Gy | Growth arrest |
| Cartilage/bone, adult | 60 Gy | Sclerosis, necrosis |

**Based on a 5% risk of late effect, 5 years after radiotherapy.*

**Table 5.1** Tissue sensitivity and late effects of radiotherapy

The earliest acute effect of superficial radiation treatment is erythema. At higher doses, such as those required for the treatment of skin malignancies and other superficial tumors, this may progress to dry and then moist desquamation. This latter is felt to be due to destruction of the basal layer of the epidermis. Following treatment, regrowth occurs from peripheral epidermal epithelial cells. There is then a transient hyperpigmentation due to stimulation of melanocytes, and then eventually the newly epithelialized skin is relatively atrophic and prone to injury from minor trauma. Late effects of high radiation dose to skin include decreased function of sweat and sebaceous glands within the treated area. Capillaries are reduced in number, predisposing to wound healing difficulty, and these and other vessels may become dilated, resulting in telangiectasias, which is part of generalized atrophy. Deeper penetrating radiation treatment, such as megavoltage photons, can cause SC fibrosis.

It should be noted that the effects on skin are dependent upon total dose, dose per fraction, and the depth of dose deposition. High doses of radiation required for epithelial tumors will result in the well-known changes described. Lower doses of radiation are generally required, for example, for hematologic malignancies, and the side effects of treatment are consequently expected to be somewhat less. Skin-sparing techniques are used in the treatment of targets residing at some depth from the skin, and thus the skin dose at the point of beam passage through the skin is only a fraction of that delivered to the target. Additionally, multiple converging beams are commonly used for such lesions, further decreasing expected skin dose.

The radiation doses commonly used for the treatment of benign proliferative diseases are much less than those used to treat malignancies. Dose per fraction may be similar, or in fact, larger to expedite treatment time and effect. The reported incidence of late effects of treatment is correspondingly lower. Even long-term results of relatively high-dose treatment of keloids and hypertrophic scars resulted in only a small incidence of skin pigmentation changes and telangiectasia, and no reported fibrosis or atrophy. This is likely related to low total dose and interfraction time for repair.

## Radiotherapy and Patient Selection

Proper patient selection for radiation treatment is especially important in the treatment of benign disease. The most common concern in treating a healthy young adult with a non-neoplastic proliferative disorder is the incidence of side effects such as wound complications, poor cosmesis, permanent normal tissue dysfunction, and the risk of inducing a secondary malignancy. For these reasons, postexcision radiotherapy is normally considered following more conventional treatments such as excision, intralesional corticosteroid injection, or pressure treatment. While certain patient populations are prone to post-treatment complications, and certain anatomical subsites are more high risk for long-term side effects, in appropriate patients, low-dose superficial radiation treatment is extremely safe and the cosmetic outcome is highly satisfactory.

Caution should be exercised in the treatment of some patients with nonmalignant systemic disorders that may increase the long-term risks associated with radiation therapy. Several studies have demonstrated that patients with active collagen vascular disease have a several-fold higher risk of late effects, particularly fibrosis. Additionally some series have implicated radiation treatments in activating systemic flares of such conditions. Interestingly, in a large retrospective series from Massachusetts General Hospital, patients with rheumatoid arthritis were the exception to this effect, and such patients had similar rates of late complications as patients without any history of collagen vascular disease. Notably, all studies demonstrating such sensitivity examined patients treated with higher dose radiation for neoplastic disorders, and there is no equivalent evidence relating to the relatively low doses used to treat benign proliferative processes. Nonetheless, caution in referring and treating such patients should be exercised.

Other systemic diseases that may increase the risk of complications of radiation treatment include hypertension, diabetes, and peripheral vascular disease. All have been shown to increase of the risk of late toxicity following irradiation, most notably post-treatment wound healing difficulties, local infection, fibrosis, and necrosis. Presumably the higher incidence of late complications in these patients is due, at least in part, to the impaired microcirculation caused by the underlying systemic disorder. A radiation-induced effect on locally released cytokines and immune complexes has also been postulated. Again, an increased risk has not been demonstrated in patients treated with low radiation doses.

There are, additionally, some patients with a genetic predisposition to complications or the development of second malignancy following radiation exposure. Defects in DNA damage repair pathways, such as those manifested in Li Fraumeni syndrome, ataxia telangiectasia, or retinoblastoma do not allow normal tissue to repair radiation-induced DNA damage as effectively, resulting in an increase in post-treatment chromosomal abnormalities and a resultant higher risk of normal tissue damage or second malignancy. Certain congenital immunodeficiencies, such as Bloom syndrome, carry a similar risk due to a similar defect in DNA damage repair. Additional inherited disorders that confer a sensitivity to x-rays are basal cell nevus syndrome (Gorlin-Goltz syndrome), Cockayne's syndrome, Down syndrome, Fanconi's anemia, Usher's syndrome, Nijmegan breakage syndrome, and Gardner's syndrome. A careful medical history will clearly identify patients in whom the risks of radiotherapy outweigh any potential benefits.

Particular caution must be exercised in the treatment of children. The same mechanism through which radiotherapy is an effective treatment for disorders of unregulated proliferation can be responsible for long-term developmental abnormalities within the radiation treatment portal. Therapeutic doses of radiation can close bone growth plates and induce organ hypoplasia, making careful treatment planning essential in such patients. These concerns are addressed by the Committee on Radiation Treatment of Benign Disease, which recommends that infants and children only be treated in very exceptional cases, and that direct irradiation of certain anatomical areas be avoided. These latter sites include areas prone to high incidence of late effects or increased risk of second malignancy (e.g. breast tissue, thyroid, bone marrow), and those in which the intrinsic sensitivity of such tissue might result in impaired function (e.g. gonads, lens). While the vast majority of such effects described in the literature are in patients treated for childhood neoplasms, late developmental effects of treatment of benign disease have been described, including breast hypoplasia following chest wall irradiation for keloid prophylaxis. This does not necessarily preclude treatment of adolescents or younger children, as the effects of radiation lie predominantly within the treatment field. Consequently, careful treatment planning to eliminate or minimize exposure to non-involved tissue can minimize the long-term risks in appropriately selected patients.

## Radiation Effects on Normal Wound Healing

Ionizing radiation can impair all stages of normal cutaneous wound healing, depending on the anatomic area irradiated, total dose, and timing. Wound healing in previously irradiated skin is impaired due to changes to both parenchymal cells and vasculature, while radiation treatment of healing wounds will have effects that depend upon the prior progress through the phases of wound healing. Potential targets of such effects include local inflammatory cells and fibroblasts.

Wound healing in previously irradiated tissue is impaired in a dose-dependent manner. The effects are mediated predominantly through fibroblasts, which have decreased proliferative capacity and permanently impaired function after radiotherapy. There is an attenuation of the normal fibroblast response to growth factor-induced chemotaxis and activation. There is both a decrease in collagen gene expression and failure of complete extracellular maturation. There is some evidence that the latter may be mediated through alterations in growth factor expression, especially transforming growth factor beta (TGF-β). The clinical consequence of this is a significant decrease in wound-bursting strength, and an increased risk of wound dehiscence. Studies of wound integrity in irradiated skin demonstrate the most significant compromise in the 3–4 weeks following injury. At later time points the strength of such wounds approaches that of wounds in unirradiated tissue.

The vasculature is also permanently altered by prior radiation. Acutely there is an increase in vascular permeability, but in the long term there is vascular stasis, occlusion, and edema of vessel walls. This results in poor vascular supply to the irradiated area, which can lead to late dermal fibrosis and resultant loss of elasticity. The loss of vascularity also predisposes to infection, and impairs the supply of monocytes and fibroblasts available for wound healing. Wounds in previously irradiated tissue are slow to heal, prone to dehisce and more readily require grafting. Grafts are more prone to breakdown, and tissue flaps more likely to fail, especially when the site of origin also lies within the radiation field.

The effects of radiation treatment on existing wounds is primarily timing dependent. Early irradiation can impair the proliferation, migration, and activation of fibroblasts, resulting in decreased collagen formation and cross-linking. Observed complications include decreased wound strength and dehiscence. In contrast, if irradiation is delayed until 3–4 weeks after wound formation, there is a much lower likelihood of complication. At least one study has demonstrated that delaying as little as 5–8 days results in a reduction of complications to the expected normal level, implying that a critical threshold of collagen formation and cross-linking has been completed. Even with such a delay, however, impaired neovascularization may occur, leading to late effects including skin atrophy, scar contraction, and fibrosis. The probability of such effects seems to be dose dependent, and thus there is a high incidence of such late complications after high-dose radiation, and a lower but significant risk following low doses such as those used in the treatment of benign proliferative processes.

## Effects of Radiotherapy on Hypertrophic Scars and Keloids

Radiotherapy is thought to prevent keloid recurrence and induce keloid regression by reversing the histopathologic changes that define hypertrophic scar or keloid formation. In both hypertrophic scars and keloids there is increased fibroblast proliferation, increased production of type I collagen, and in keloids there is enhanced fibroblast activation in response to growth factors. Studies of the effects of radiation on normal wound healing have demonstrated an inhibition of fibroblast proliferative capacity for treatment administered during the inflammatory phase, consistent with clinical data that suggests optimal efficacy of radiotherapy when it is delivered within 24–48 hours of keloid excision. Likewise, irradiated fibroblasts in normal tissue have attenuated collagen production, and diminished activation and chemotaxis in response to growth factors. Radiation treatment also induces cell death in some portion of the fibroblast population, diminishing the reservoir of cells available for proliferation and collagen synthesis.

A second postulated mechanism of action of radiation in the prevention of benign proliferative disease relates to monocytes and their sensitivity to radiation-induced programmed cell death (apoptosis). Early in the inflammatory phase of wound healing, a decrease in the population of monocytes would be expected to impair growth factor induction of fibroblast migration, activation and proliferation. This potential mechanism is also supported by the successful use of radiation treatment in the early post-excision interval (Fig. 5.6).

## Clinical evidence

There is a single randomized trial of post-excision radiotherapy for keloids. A total of 31 patients at Beth Israel Hospital were treated after excision of keloids with pathologic confirmation of the diagnosis. They were randomized to corticosteroid injection or local radiotherapy, and 28 patients completed their assigned treatment. Of the 16 patients treated with radiation there were two recurrences (12.5%) vs. four of the 12 patients treated with steroid injection (33%). Due to the small sample size, this difference was not statistically significant, but the authors also noted that patients in the radiation arm were more likely to complete their adjuvant therapy.

The remainder of the clinical evidence suggesting that radiation is effective for prevention of keloid recurrence is retrospective, and consists of predominantly single institution experiences. Selected reports are summarized in Table 5.2. Inalsingh et al reported the results of treating 501 patients with radiation, though not all lesions were excised prior to therapy. They were treated with 4 Gy monthly, with one to five fractions. Of all patients treated, 76% had complete regression of keloids at the 2-year follow up.

Borok et al reported on the treatment of 375 keloids in 250 patients, the majority of which were excised prior to radiation. There were only nine significant recurrences (2.4%), of which seven were in patients who had subsequent ear lobe piercing. There were no reported wound complications. The authors used a variety of fractionation schemes, all utilizing kilovoltage photons. Their recommendation was a total dose of 12 Gy, administered in three fractions with the first treatment immediately following excision. This is one of the more common schedules in use today.

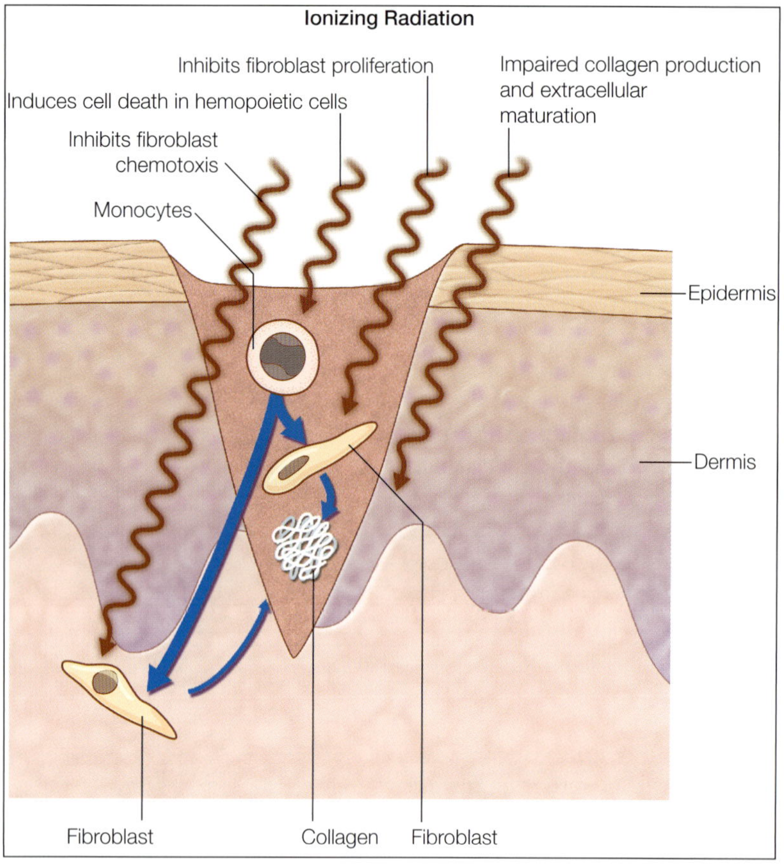


**Fig. 5.6** Radiotherapy targets in normal and abnormal wound healing. Ionizing radiation affects several targets in the wound-healing process. Radiation treatment induces apoptosis in inflammatory cells, and impairs fibroblast proliferation and function

| Clinical Evidence for Radiotherapy in Keloid Prophylaxis | | | |
|---|---|---|---|
| **Study author** | **No. patients** | **Follow up** | **Freedom from recurrence** |
| Sclafani | 31 | 1 year | 77.5% |
| Inalsingh | 501 | 2 years | 76% |
| Borok | 250 | <1 year | 97.6% |
| Lo | 199 | 3 years | 82%* |
| Kovalic | 75 | 10 years | 73% |
| Doornbos | 218 | 1 year | 90%* |
| **For patients treated beyond threshold dose.* | | | |

**Table 5.2** Clinical evidence for radiotherapy in keloid prophylaxis

Lo reported the Lahey Clinic experience of 354 keloids treated in 199 patients. A total of 174 lesions were treated post excision with a single fraction of electron irradiation. With doses of 9 Gy or greater, the control rate was 82% at a median follow up of 35 months. A total of 63 patients treated without prior excision had significantly higher recurrence rates, though regression of disease was noted in 48% of lesions.

One of the longest reported follow-up studies is from Kovalic et al, with 113 keloids in 75 patients followed for a median of 9.75 years. Patients were treated after excision, with the most common treatment schedule being 12 Gy over 3 days. There was a 73% control rate, with risk factors for recurrence being size greater than 2 cm, male gender, and prior treatment. No complications were noted.

Treatment decisions are, of course, made on an individual basis. In terms of type of ionizing radiation, the lack of availability of an orthovoltage treatment machine, for example, may dictate electrons as the sole treatment modality. Anatomic contours, target size, proximity and tissue depth of surrounding critical structures, and patient positioning may make one modality more advantageous than another. The goal is to achieve dose homogeneity to the target while limiting the dose to underlying normal tissue. Bolus, a tissue-density material, may be used to increase the skin surface dose and decrease the depth dose. In some clinical situations, such as earlobes, high-energy photons can be directed in an anterior/posterior direction to treat the entire thickness of a structure while keeping normal tissue out of the treatment field. Thoughtful treatment planning is required to both maximize clinical efficacy and minimize potential treatment morbidity, and consultation with an experienced radiation therapist prior to planned excision is essential since treatment is often initiated within 24–48 hours of excision.

## Expected Acute and Late Sequelae of Radiation Treatment

High-dose superficial radiation, such as is required for the treatment of superficial malignancies, can result in significant acute and long-term morbidity. Erythema develops early during the treatment course, followed by dry and moist desquamation. Re-population of the epidermis occurs following cessation of treatment, but the newly formed skin is atrophic, sensitive to trauma, and prone to wound healing complications. Late effects include formation of telangiectasias due to dilation of capillaries, hypopigmentation, permanent alopecia, loss of sebaceous and sweat gland function, and SC fibrosis (Box 5.1).

Lower doses, such as those appropriate for treatment of hypertrophic scars or keloids, have dramatically fewer such side effects. During or immediately following treatment there may be erythema at the higher range of appropriate doses, but more commonly there are no noticeable effects. Multiple series have reported no complications in the healing of the excision wound. There is a relative paucity of data regarding other local late effects, though the most common appears to be hypopigmentation, and the incidence is less than 5–10%. A similarly

**Dose-Dependent Clinical Effects of Radiotherapy Treatment to the Skin**

Acute effects
- Erythema
- Dry desquamation
- Moist desquamation

Late effects
- Hypopigmentation
- Hyperpigmentation
- Telangiectasia (atrophy)
- Permanent epilation
- Subcutaneous fibrosis
- Necrosis

**Box 5.1** Dose-dependent clinical effects of radiotherapy treatment to the skin low incidence of scar contraction or fibrosis would be expected. Permanent, localized alopecia would not be expected at these doses.

One of the greatest areas of concern in regard to irradiating a non-neoplastic process in an otherwise healthy young adult is the long-term risk of second malignancy. The low doses used for such treatment may be paradoxically more likely to be carcinogenic than higher doses. The former are felt to induce sublethal DNA damage, leading to propagation of mutation, while the latter is cytotoxic. Although reported series of keloid irradiation report no carcinogenesis, the follow up of these studies tends to be in the range of 1–8 years. In contrast, the expected latency of radiation-induced malignancy would be in the range of 10–30 years. Several case reports are available of patients who subsequently developed a suspicious malignancy within or near the previous radiation portal after treatment of keloids. One male patient developed thyroid cancer 8 years after radiation directed at his chin, and two women developed breast cancer 20 and 30 years following chest wall irradiation. One of these breast cancer patients had underlying breast hypoplasia stemming from high-dose irradiation during development, and the second had two adjacent metachronous primaries within or near her treatment field. These anecdotal reports are cause for concern, especially when considering treatment of radiosensitive areas such as breast and thyroid, but given the large number of patients treated, the incidence of such carcinogenesis is clearly quite low.

## Recommendations

A number of retrospective reports, and a single, albeit small, randomized trial, have examined the efficacy of localized, low-dose irradiation for the prevention of recurrence of hypertrophic scars or keloids. Radiation treatment after excision is consistently noted to be one of the most safe and effective treatment strategies. In appropriately selected patients, it is extremely safe both in terms of acute and late morbidity, and well tolerated. Most patients treated with radiation are referred after having failed more conservative management strategies, and this may be due to concern over long-term risks of radiotherapy such as poor cosmesis or the induction of secondary malignancy. Although the latter are reported only anecdotally, caution should be exercised in the routine referral of patients for treatment of a benign proliferative process with predominantly cosmetic implications, and initial trials of more conservative therapy are appropriate. Infants and young children should be treated only in exceptional circumstances, and radiosensitive areas such as the breast and thyroid should be avoided. In all patients, the treating radiation therapist should minimize dose to uninvolved normal structures.

The most common treatment regimen incorporates kilovoltage photon or megavoltage electron external beam radiation. The total dose of 10–15 Gy should be delivered over several days. The treatment is often initiated within 24–48 hours of excision, though the clinical data to support this are sparse. The complexity of treatment planning, and importance of timing, makes early referral (i.e. pre-excision) essential so that potential risks and benefits can be discussed with the patient in detail. A significant decrease in recurrence following radiotherapy is expected in 80–90% of patients. Radiation of unexcised hypertrophic scars and keloids can be performed in patients in whom such excision is not practicable. The expected efficacy is significantly lower, and this is not routinely recommended.

## Further Reading

Borok TL, Bray M, Sinclair I, et al 1988 Role of ionizing irradiation for 393 keloids. International Journal of Radiation, Oncology, Biology, Physics 15:865–870

Doornbos JF, Stoffel TJ, Hass AC, et al 1990 The role of kilovoltage irradiation in the treatment of keloids. International Journal of Radiation, Oncology, Biology, Physics 18:833–839

Emami B, Lyman J, Brown A, et al 1991 Tolerance of normal tissue to therapeutic irradiation. International Journal of Radiation, Oncology, Biology, Physics 21:109–122

Inalsingh CH 1974 An experience in treating five hundred and one patients with keloids. Johns Hopkins Medical Journal 134:284–290

Kovalic JJ, Perez CA 1989 Radiation therapy following keloidectomy: a 20-year experience. International Journal of Radiation, Oncology, Biology, Physics 17:77–80

Lo TC, Seckel BR, Salzman FA, Wright KA 1990 Single-dose electron beam irradiation in treatment and prevention of keloids and hypertrophic scars. Radiotherapy and Oncology 19:267–272

Rubin P, Soni A, Williams JP 1999 The molecular and cellular biologic basis for the radiation treatment of benign proliferative diseases. Seminars in Radiation and Oncology 9:203–214

Sclafani AP, Gordon L, Chadha M, Romo T III 1996 Prevention of earlobe keloid recurrence with postoperative corticosteroid injections versus radiation therapy: a randomized, prospective study and review of the literature. Dermatologic Surgery 22:569–574

Tibbs MK 1997 Wound healing following radiation therapy: a review. Radiotherapy and Oncology 42:99–106

# 6 Laser-induced Repigmentation of Scars

*Roy G. Geronemus, Galen H. Fisher*

## Introduction

One reason that scars stand out from the surrounding normal skin is because they are often a different color. Color changes associated with scars include erythema, temporary hyperpigmentation and hypopigmentation. Erythema is typically associated with immature scars and treatment of this is discussed elsewhere within this volume. This chapter will focus on the use of ultraviolet B (UVB) in the treatment of hypopigmented scars.

## Causes of Hypopigmentation

Mature scars often appear hypopigmented compared to surrounding normal skin. The most common explanation of the hypopigmentation is that the areas affected have decreased melanocyte numbers compared to the surrounding skin. However, recent immunohistochemical analyses by Velangi et al demonstrated preservation of epidermal melanocytes within scar tissue. Their findings raise the possibility that hypopigmentation of scars may not simply be due to a decrease in melanocyte number but rather an optical effect due to alterations in collagen and microvasculature. These studies also laid the theoretical foundation for using lasers and phototherapy devices that emit in the UVB spectrum to repigment scars.

## Use of UVB Lasers for Repigmentation

Light energy in the UVB spectrum has been shown to be useful for inducing repigmentation of hypopigmented scars, striae albae, $CO_2$ laser resurfacing-induced leukoderma, as well as laser tattoo removal-induced leukoderma. UVB has successfully been used to repigment hypopigmented scars in patients of all skin types (I–VI).

### Candidates for UVB laser treatment

Patients who are good candidates for UVB-induced repigmentation include those with hypopigmented scars who do not have any contraindications to UVB phototherapy. Contraindications include: patients with a photosensitive genodermatosis, with photoaggravated disease (e.g. systemic lupus erythematosis [SLE]), with a history of numerous skin cancers, with a history of radiation therapy within the area to be treated with UVB, with organ transplants that require immunosuppression, and on photosensitizing medicines. It is also important that the patient understands that multiple treatments will be necessary and that maintenance therapy will be required to maintain the response.

## Expected benefits

Based on the current authors' experience using a 308 nm Excimer laser, they feel that the following benefits can be expected from UVB treatment (they obtained similar results with Lumenis' ReLume, a hand-held UVB phototherapy device [Fig. 6.1]). They saw an average of 62% improvement in patients treated for repigmentation of hypopigmented scars after nine biweekly treatments (Fig. 6.2). It is important to note that this repigmentation is not permanent and fades back to baseline within 5–6 months for most patients (Fig. 6.2). They did observe that the induced pigment was more stable in patients with darker skin tones (III–VI).

In general, this treatment is well tolerated and safe. The treatment itself is painless and requires no preparation of the area other than removal of any topical agents that might absorb the 308 nm Excimer laser. Side effects that might be encountered following 308 nm Excimer laser-induced repigmentation of scars include erythema, blister formation, local irritation, photoallergic response, and hyperpigmentation, all of which are rare. There is also a theoretical side effect of induction of actinic damage and possibly induction of nonmelanoma skin cancer. At this time there have not been any studies that adequately quantify

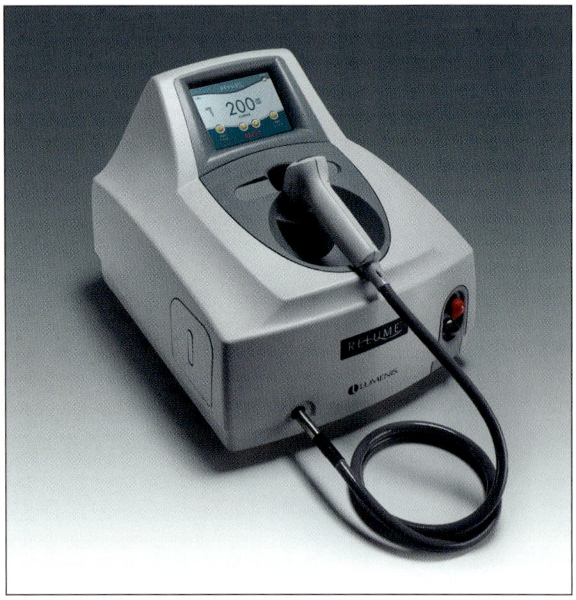


**Fig. 6.1** A hand-held UVB-emitting laser. Courtesy of Relume

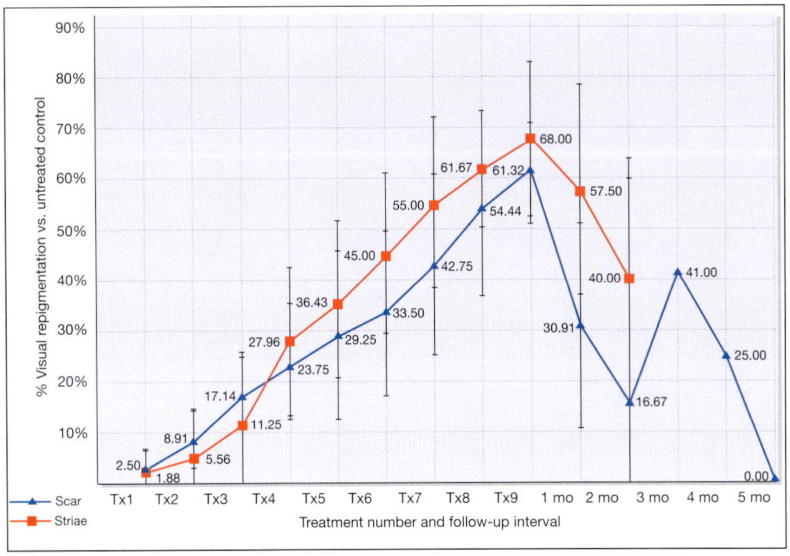


**Fig. 6.2** Mean percentage of pigmentation correction of treated sites as assessed visually by three blinded observers. Pigmentation of the treated site was visually compared to a matched, untreated, control site. The x-axis indicates treatment number (administered weekly) and follow-up interval (monthly) (Courtesy of Alexiades-Armenakas et al 2004)

the carcinogeneic risk from this type of UVB exposure, however the concern should be minimal given that the cumulative dose of UVB is low.

## Treatment strategy

The treatment strategy is to first establish a given patient's minimal erythematous dose (MED). This is done by applying a series of test spots to thc torso or volar forcarm in 50 mJ/cm$^2$ increments ranging from 100–300 mJ/cm$^2$. MED is evaluated 24 hours following administration of the test spots. The first treatment is applied at a dose of 50 mJ/cm$^2$ less than the MED. Treatments are administered on a biweekly basis. The dose is held at the same level until it no longer results in clinical improvement or erythema. At that point the treatment dose is increased by 50 mJ/cm$^2$ per treatment until a clinical response or erythema is seen. There are no special postoperative care instructions that need to be given besides advising the patient to avoid direct sun exposure to the area, as this might result in too great a dose being administered to the area. Patients are treated on a biweekly basis until the desired clinical endpoint is reached (Fig. 6.3 A–D and 6.4 A–B). In the current authors' experience this usually requires between 7–10 treatments. It is important to shield adjacent nonscar tissue from UVB light to prevent the adjacent skin from becoming hyperpigmented. This shielding can be done with an opaque material such as cardboard or tongue depressors, or UVB impermeable plexiglas can be used. One advantage of cardboard is that it can be used to make a

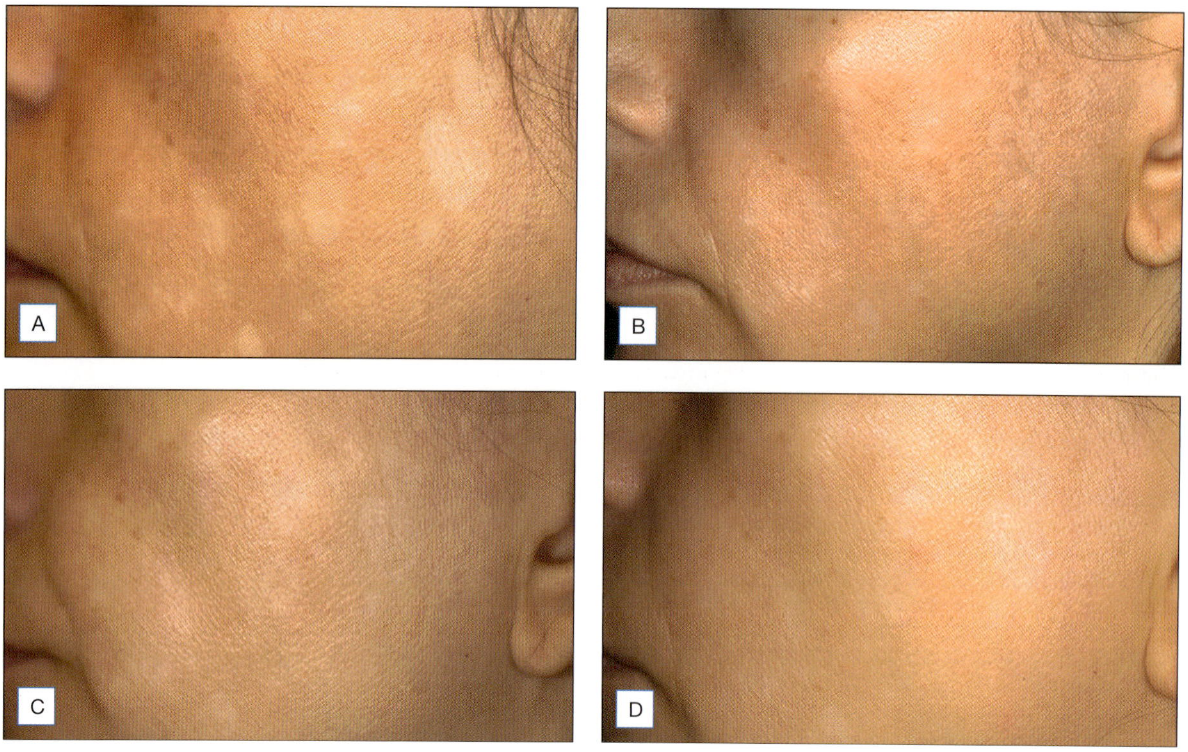


**Fig. 6.3** Hypopigmented scars treated with 308 nm Excimer laser. At baseline (**A**) prominent hypopigmented scars are seen on the left cheek, following five treatments (**B**) there is significant repigmentation; 2 months following cessation of treatment there is some dimunition in pigment (**C**) and by 6 months follow-up (**D**) the scars appear similar to baseline. (Photo 6.3a–d courtesy of Alexiades-Armenakas et al 2004)

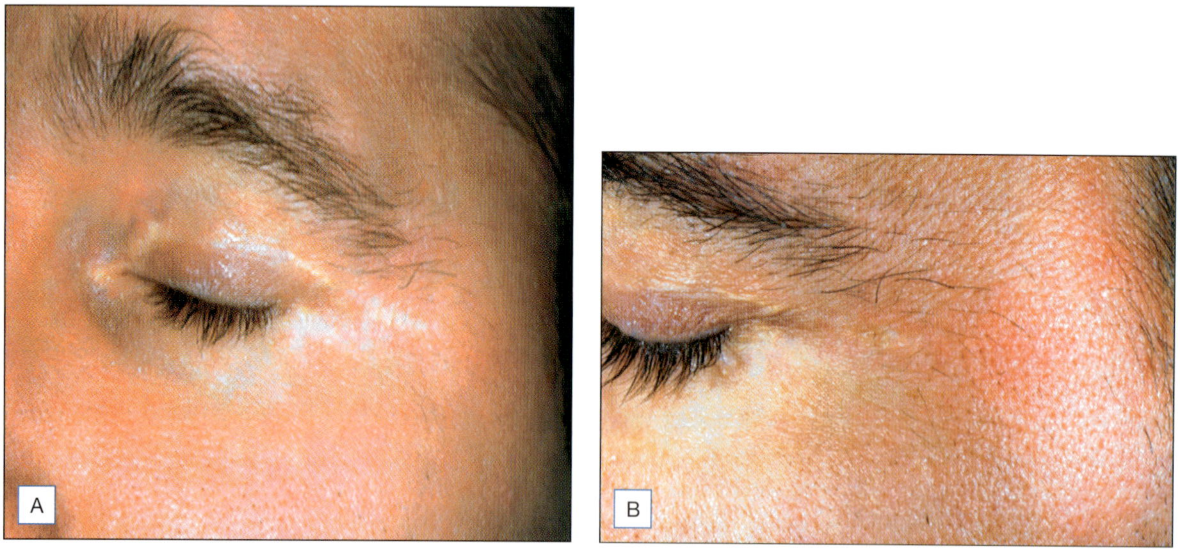


**Fig. 6.4** (**A**) Photograph of postblepharoplasty hypopigmented scar on left upper lid extending lateral to the left lateral commissure. (**B**) Photograph showing repigmentation of the blepharoplasty scar following nine treatments with a hand-held UVB-emitting phototherapy device

custom cut-out for each patient's scar (Fig. 6.5). The cardboard template can be saved in the patient's chart for reuse at each visit. They do not advocate using sunscreens to shield the surrounding skin as this method is likely to result in inadvertent shielding of the scar and possibly contamination of the optics of the laser with sunscreen. Maintenance treatments are needed approximately every 1–2 months for patients with types I–II and slightly less frequently for patients with darker skin tones (Fig. 6.6, Box 6.1).

## Available devices

There are currently two devices that are convenient sources of hand-held UVB energy. The first is the 308 nm Excimer laser and the second is the Lumenis' Relume UVB hand-held phototherapy device, which emits over the entire UVB spectrum of 290–320 nM. Both devices have been used to successfully and safely induce pigmentation within scars. The current authors are not aware of significant advantages of one UVB-emitting device over the other.

### Overview of UVB-Induced Repigmentation Treatment Protocol

- Establish MED
- Begin first treatment at 50 mJ/cm$^2$ less than MED
- If no clinical response or erythema, increase by 50 mJ/cm$^2$
- Treat on a biweekly basis until desired level of pigment is induced
- Maintenance therapy every 2 months as needed

**Box 6.1** Overview of UVB-induced repigmentation treatment protocol

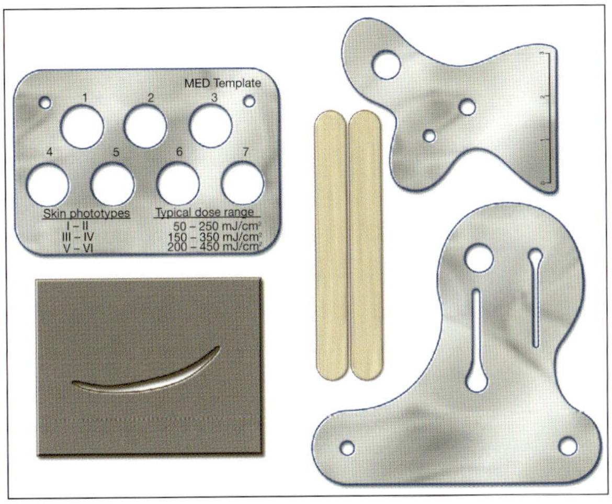


**Fig. 6.5** Commercially available and homemade UVB shields. These facilitate selective treatment of only the hypopigmented scar and prevent hyperpigmentation of surrounding skin

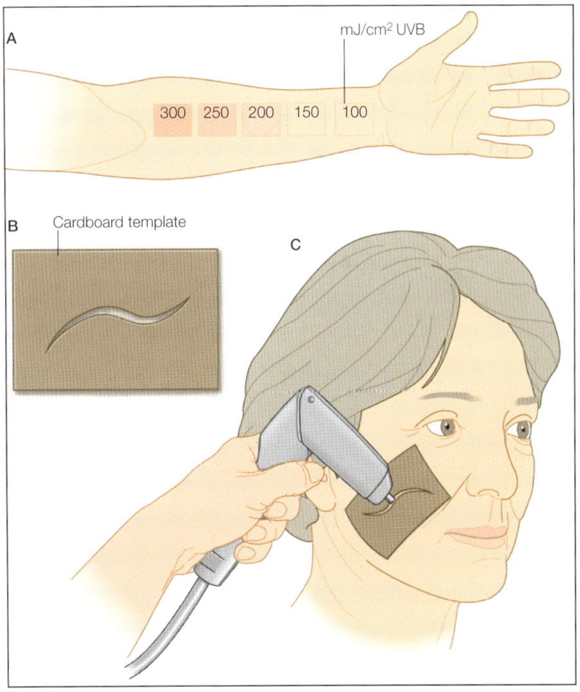


**Fig. 6.6** Laser repigmentation of scars. As shown in **A**, the first step is to determine the patient's minimal erythema dose (MED). This is typically done on a sun-protected area such as the volar forearm. Increasing doses of UVB are given from 100–300 J in increments of 50 J. Once the MED has been determined, a template is created to protect the normally pigmented skin surrounding the treatment area (**B**). Then, as shown in **C**, the scar is treated on a biweekly basis and the energy is increased by 50 J per treatment if neither erythema nor clinical improvement are noted

## Alternate therapies

In addition to UVB-induced repigmentation of scars, theoretically a surgical approach that is currently in use for vitiligo could be used: melanocyte transfer. The current authors have not tried this approach for scar repigmentation but would like to present it here as it could theoretically prove useful in patients seeking a more permanent repigmentation. However, the studies of Velangi et al do raise the question of whether or not the hypopigmentation of scars in fact represents a decrease in melanocytes within the area of scar.

### *Melanocyte transplantation*

Melanocyte transplantation has been used for treatment of recalcitrant vitiligo. There are four main variations of melanocyte transplantation that are currently in use for treatment of vitiligo: punch grafting, suction or psoralen plus UVA (PUVA) blister grafting, ultrathin split-thickness skin grafting, and transfer of cultured melanocytes. Given that access to melanocyte culturing is likely limited for most practitioners and that published reports of success with cultured melanocytes have varied considerably, only the first three of these approaches will be briefly discussed.

### *Punch micrografting*

Punch micrografting has been used to restore pigment islands to areas of vitiligo. The melanocytes that are contained within the islands can then spread out into the surrounding vitiliginous skin and potentially repigment the entire vitiliginous patch over time. The technique is quite simple. A 1.5–2 mm trephine is used to remove plugs of epidermis and SC tissue to create recipient sites within the area to be repigmented. Into the recipient sites are placed full-thickness skin plugs of the exact same diameter from nonvitiliginous skin (Fig. 6.7). It is best to harvest the donor plugs from a cosmetically inconspicuous area that best matches the recipient site in skin texture. The plugs can either be sutured in place or preferably the area can simply be dressed with an occlusive dressing for 1 week. Potential complications include infection, bleeding, scaring and nontotal repigmentation that produces a mottled or cobblestoned appearance. This procedure should be used with caution in patients with a history of keloids.

### *Epidermal blister roofs*

The second approach is the use of epidermal blister roofs (Fig. 6.8). This approach requires the use of either a vacuum-generating device or PUVA to generate blisters. Recent reports have shown that a simple three-way stopcock coupled with a 50 ml syringe and a manometer can be used to inexpensively and reliably generate suction blisters. The roof of the blisters are harvested and placed in a dish of sterile saline or on saline-soaked sterile gauze while the recipient site is prepared. The recipient site is prepared by either laser ablation of the epidermis

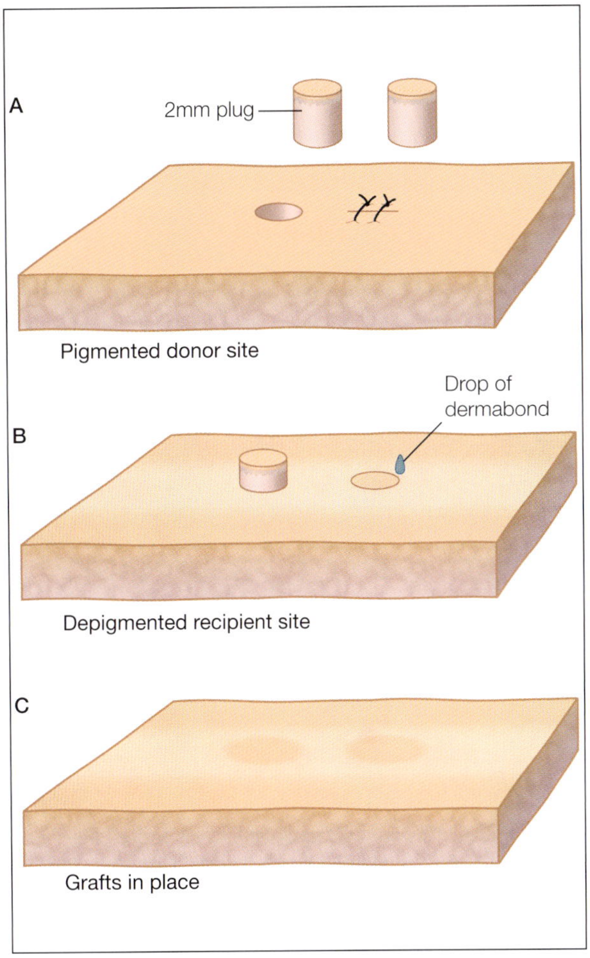


**Fig. 6.7** The process of punch grafting. **A**, depicts the harvesting of 2 mm plugs of normally pigmented skin. As shown in **B**, these are transferred to donor sites created within the area of hypopigmentation. Once these sites heal there will be islands of normal pigmentation at the sites of punch graft transfer, **C**. Over time the melanocytes will spread a few millimeters into the surrounding area

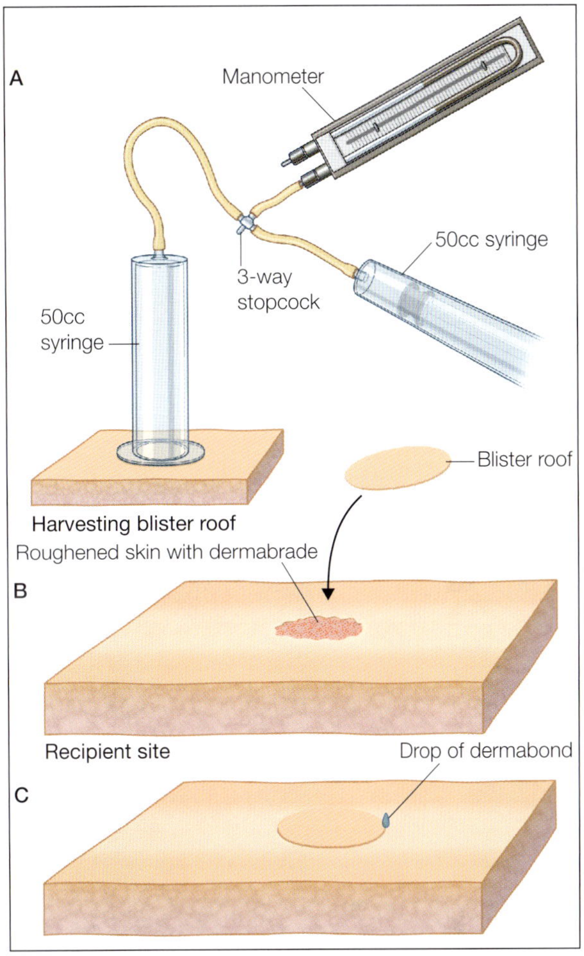


**Fig. 6.8** Suction or PUVA blister grafting. The first step is to generate a suction blister. As is shown in **A**, negative pressure is applied to normally pigmented skin (to enhance the effect the site can be pretreated with PUVA to facilitate blister formation). As is shown in **B**, the recipient site is prepared by de-epithelialization (either by suction blister or dermabrasion). The roof of the donor site suction blister is then secured to the recipient site and allowed to heal. As shown in **C**, this will result in an island of normally pigmented skin

with a $CO^2$ or erbium:yttrium–aluminum–garnet (Er:YAG) laser or by standard dermabrasion techniques. The blister roof graft is then placed over the prepared recipient site and held in place using an occlusive dressing for 1 week. Complications of this approach include hyperpigmentation of the donor site as well as graft failure. In a review of the literature there were no reports of donor site scarring. The third approach to melanocyte transfer is the use of ultrathin split-thickness skin grafts: **flip-top** grafting (Figs 6.9 and 6.10). The success of this approach depends on the use of ultrathin grafts (< 0.001 mm in thickness). The main disadvantage of this approach is one of technical

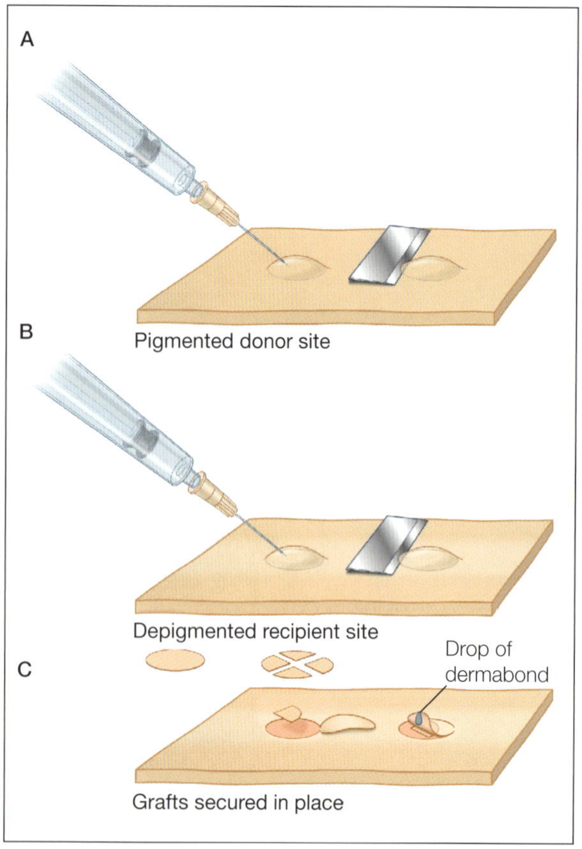


**Fig. 6.9** 'Flip-top' pigment transfer. (**A**) shows the harvesting of donor skin. Local anesthesia is used to raise a wheal of skin, from which a thin sliver of normally pigmented epithelium is shaved. (**B**) shows the preparation of the recipient site with a nearly identical process except that the thin sliver of skin is left attached at one edge to create an ultrathin 'flip-top' flap. (**C**) shows the harvested 5 mm diameter graft subdivided into 4-5 evenly sized pieces before being placed in the recipient sites and secured in place dermal side down beneath the 'flip-top' with dermabond

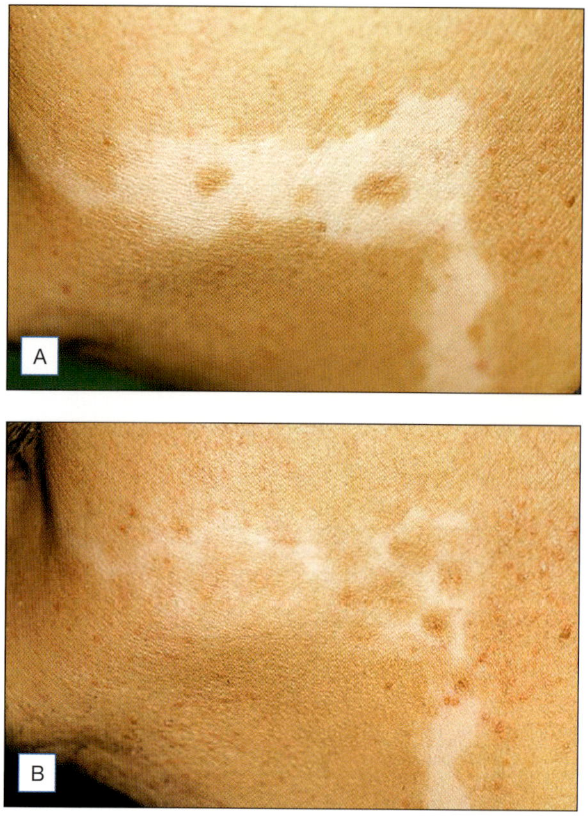


**Fig. 6.10** Flip-top pigment transplantation treatment of vitiligo. (**A**) Patient shown after receiving two grafts in the area of vitiligo. (**B**) 5 months after the placement of nine grafts (Photo courtesy of McGovern et al 1999)

difficulty in harvesting the graft. Postoperative care requires that the graft be held in place with an occlusive dressing.

In addition to using UVB to induce repigmentation of scars, the current authors have recently seen some tantalizing but paradoxical results with fractional photothermolysis (Fraxel laser, Reliant technologies, Palo-Alto, CA). Fractional photothermolysis is a mid-infrared, 1550 nm laser which induces epidermal and dermal remodeling by creating microscopic columns of thermal damage called **microthermal zones** (MTZs). Each MTZ has a diameter of approximately 50 μm (slightly more at higher energies). The density of the MTZs can be varied but is usually kept at 2000 per $cm^2$ per treatment. At this point, the results they have seen with using fractional photothermolysis to treat pigment abnormalities can be best described as pigment normalization. They have noted that when areas of tattoo-removal laser-induced leukoderma are treated, the area becomes more pigmented. However, when they treat areas of facial hyperpigmentation secondary to melasma or photo-induced lentignes, these areas become less pigmented and are 'normalized' relative to the surrounding skin. They do not see clinical evidence of hyperpigmentation of normal skin. At this time they are in the process of elucidating the variables dictating the clinical response as well as durability of the clinical response.

## Further Reading


Alexiades-Armenakas MR, Bernstein LJ, Friedman PM, Geronemus RG 2004 The safety and efficacy of the 308-nm excimer laser for pigment correction of hypopigmented scars and striae alba. Archives of Dermatology 140:955–960

Arroyo MP, Tift L 2003 Vitiligo therapy: where are we now? Journal of Drugs in Dermatology 2:404–408

Falabella R 2003 Surgical treatment of vitiligo: why, when and how. Journal of the European Academy of Dermatology and Venereology 17:518–520

Friedman PM, Geronemus RG 2001 Use of the 308-nm excimer laser for postresurfacing leukoderma. Archives of Dermatology 137:824–825

Gupta S, Shroff S, Gupta S 1999 Modified technique of suction blistering for epidermal grafting in vitiligo. International Journal of Dermatology 38:306–309

Issa CM, Rehder J, Taube MB 2003 Melanocyte transplantation for the treatment of vitiligo: effects of different surgical techniques. European Journal of Dermatology 13:34–39

McGovern TW, Bolognia J, Leffell DJ 1999 Flip-top pigment transplantation: a novel transplantation procedure for the treatment of depigmentation. Archives of Dermatology 135:1305-1307

van Geel N, Ongenae K, Naeyaert JM 2001 Surgical techniques for vitiligo: a review. Dermatology 202:162–166

Velangi SS, Rees JL 2001 Why are scars pale? An immunohistochemical study indicating preservation of melanocyte number and function in surgical scars. ACTA Dermato-Venereologica 81:326–328

# 7 Special Considerations in Approach to Treatment and Management of Scars in African-Americans and Other Populations More at Risk

*A. Paul Kelly*

## Introduction

Patients often present with itchy and/or painful ugly scars and want to make sure these raised lesions are not cancer. They have keloids, which are benign skin growths of variable size and shape resulting from excessive connective tissue response, in genetically predisposed individuals, to skin trauma. There are, however, spontaneous keloids, which arise without a history of previous trauma, most commonly located over the sternum. The incidence of keloids is highest in black-skinned individuals (Box 7.1) and lowest in Caucasians, while the incidence in those of Asian and Latino origin falls somewhere in between. The ratio of black individuals compared to Caucasians ranges from 5:1–16:1, yet once keloids develop, the recurrence ratio after surgical removal is the same for all races (Box 7.1). Earlobe keloids following ear piercing are the most common, but if they occur without keloids located in other anatomic areas, they offer no clue to the likelihood of the same person forming keloids elsewhere. They are usually located on the posterior lobe (Fig. 7.1). When the anterior and posterior lobes are involved, the posterior lesion is usually larger (Fig. 7.2). Other times, keloids wrap around the lobe, making surgery difficult (Fig. 7.3). Other common areas for keloid formation are the anterior and lateral neck (Fig. 7.4), chest (Fig. 7.5), abdomen (Fig. 7.6) and upper back. Keloids rarely

**Risk Factors for Keloid Recurrence**

- Family history of keloids
- Infected operative site
- Midchest, shoulder
- Thermal or chemical burn
- Tension on scar
- Dark skin

**Box 7.1** Risk factors for keloid recurrence

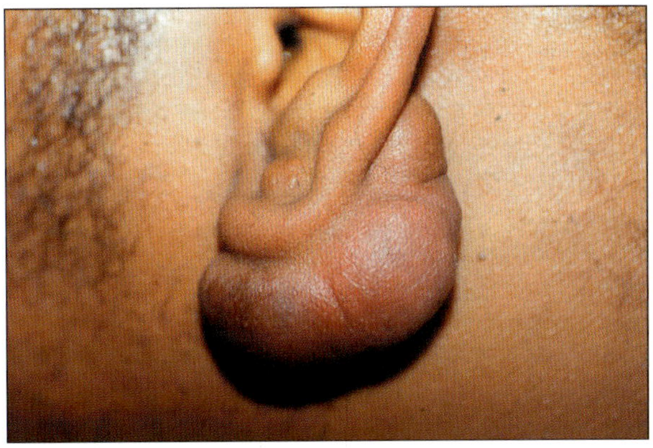

**Fig. 7.1** Keloid on posterior ear lobe

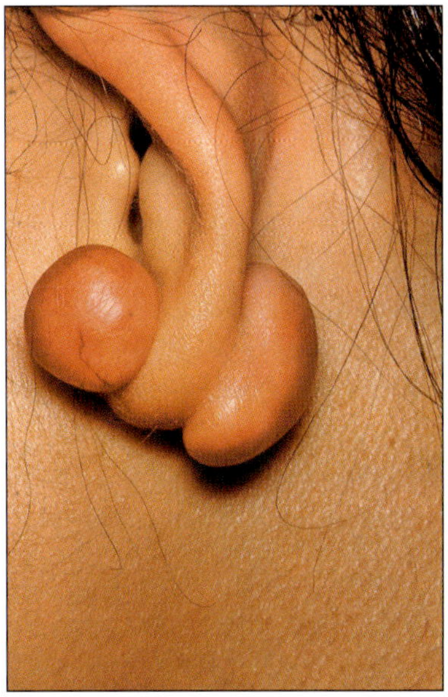

**Fig. 7.2** Dumbbell keloid on anterior and posterior earlobe with larger posterior lesions

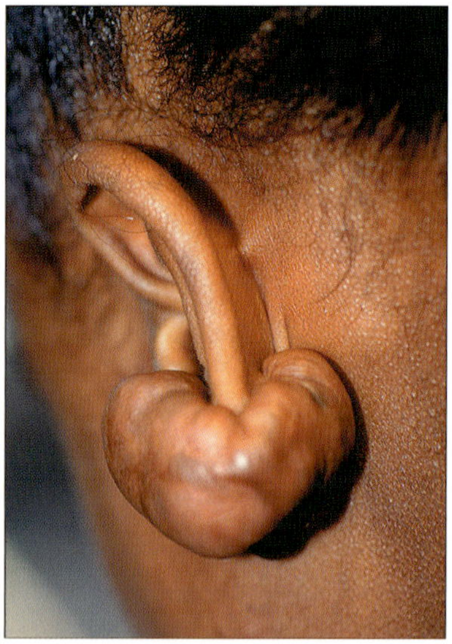

**Fig. 7.3** Wraparound keloid on left ear lobe

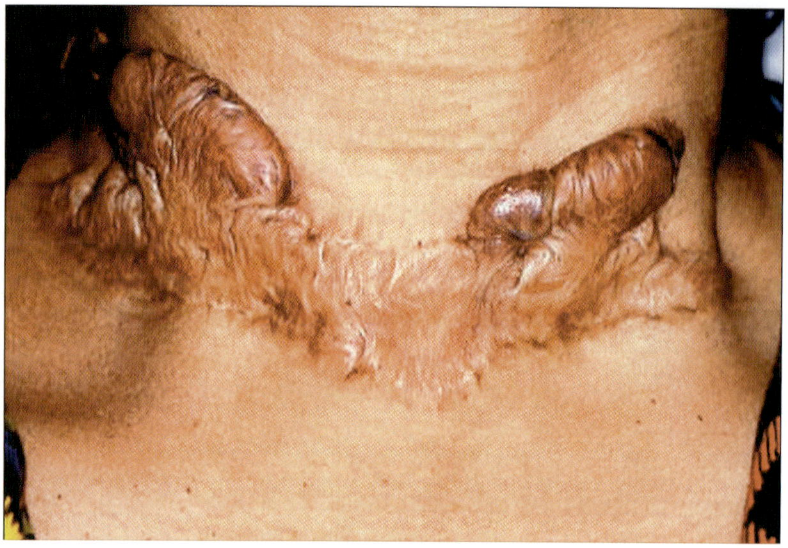

**Fig. 7.4** Keloid on anterior and lateral neck

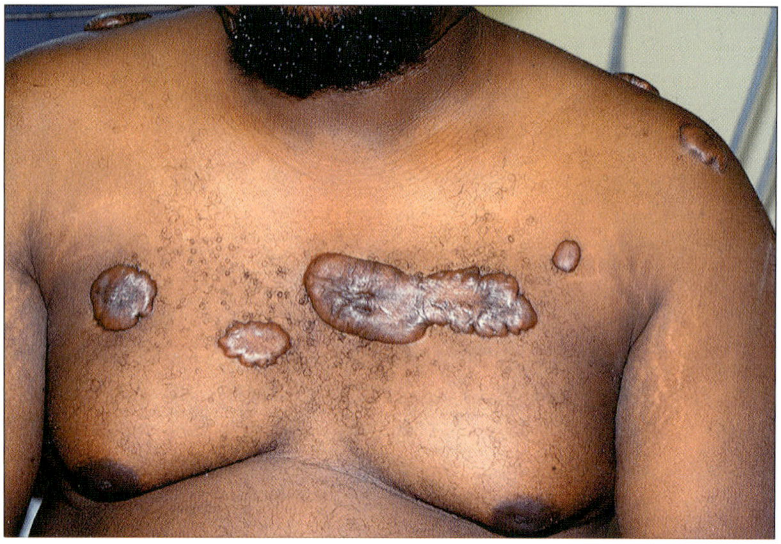

**Fig. 7.5** Keloids on chest

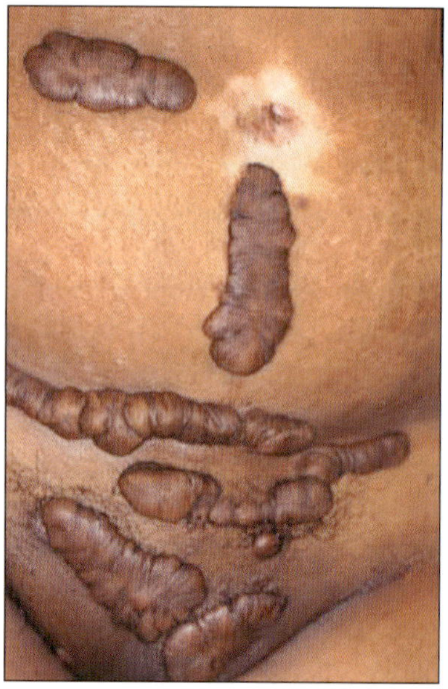

**Fig. 7.6** Keloids on abdomen plus area of hypopigmentation where umbilical area was injected with 40 mg/cc of triamcinolone acetonide

occur on the hands, feet, scalp and axillae (Fig. 7.7). Except for patients who develop keloids secondary to chemical or thermal burns and children with chickenpox, most keloids occur in the second and third decades of life. There is no gender difference in the incidence of keloids except for those secondary to ear piercing, which are more common in females; however, with the relatively recent fashion of males wearing one earring, the incidence of men with ear lobe keloids is increasing. Keloids may be asymptomatic but are usually pruritic and may also be painful and have a burning or warm sensation.

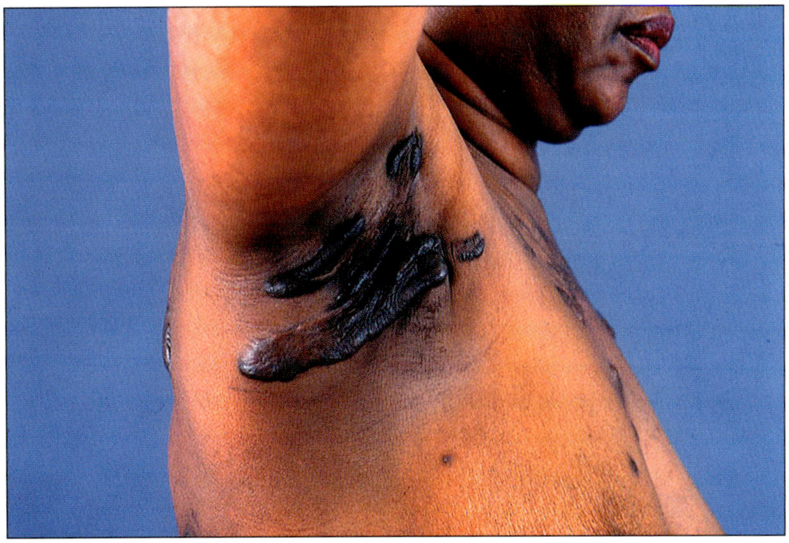

**Fig. 7.7** Keloids on right axilla

| Clinical Differences between Keloids and Hypertrophic Scars | |
|---|---|
| **Keloids** | **Hypertrophic scars** |
| Invade clinically normal skin | Limited to traumatized areas |
| May continue growing for the patient's lifetime | Usually regress spontaneously in 12–18 months |
| Often resistant to therapy | Respond to therapy |
| Erythematous borders indicate continued growth and may grow for a patient's lifetime | Rarely grow after 2–3 months |
| Pruritic, painful, burning | Usually asymptomatic |

**Table 7.1** Clinical differences between keloids and hypertrophic scars

The differential diagnosis between early keloids and hypertrophic scars may be difficult. Clinically, hypertrophic scars are limited to traumatized areas, respond to therapy, and regress spontaneously in 12–18 months. Keloids, on the other hand, invade clinically normal skin adjacent to the traumatized area and have a poor response to therapy (Table. 7.1).

Before initiating therapy in known keloids formers, the physician should be aware of preventive measures. Ear piercing and nonessential cosmetic surgery, etc. (face lifts, breast reduction or augmentation, tummy tucks, or tattoos) should be withheld. All surgical wounds should be closed with normal tension, incisions should not cross joint spaces, mid-chest incisions should be avoided, and incisions should follow the skin creases whenever possible. The same holds true if the patients' parents or siblings have keloids.

## Keloid Therapeutic Gems

Before discussing racial and ethnic differences in keloid therapy, a few therapeutic gems should be discussed. Prior to injecting intralesional steroids the patient should apply EMLA (Rx AstraZeneca, Wilmington, DE) Cream, L.M.X4. (Rx Ferndale, Ferndale, MI) topical anesthetic cream thickly on the keloid and wait 1 hour before injecting. Inject into the papillary dermis (this is where collagenase is produced). Insert the needle a little deeper and inject as the needle is slowly withdrawn, until the dermal epidermal plane is reached, where the triamcinolone acetonide goes in easily. Inject with a small-bore needle, 27–30 gauge, because larger needles sometimes behave as a biopsy punch and become clogged with keloid tissue, making it impossible to inject. This is especially true with the early injections when the keloid is still hard. Injections should be given every third week and not started until 2–3 weeks after the sutures have been removed, or the postoperative site may dehisce. Although the current authors have never encountered adrenal suppression with larger doses, the maximum amount of triamcinolone acetonide 40 mg/cc per session is $1\frac{1}{2}$ cc. Higher doses may be safe but they have never had a problem with $1\frac{1}{2}$ cc of 40 mg/cc triamcinolone. Also, at the time of surgical removal a half-and-half mixture of triamcinolone 40 mg/cc and 2% lidocaine with epinephrine is used for anesthesia. If injecting is still too painful or difficult, the perilesional area of the keloid should be injected with 1% lidocaine. This enables painless keloid injections. The steroid will cause a delay in wound healing so sutures should be left in for 2–3 weeks, except for the face, where, for 10 days is sufficient.

Each time a patient with keloids comes for therapy, the lesions should be checked for a partial or complete erythematous border (Fig. 7.8); if this is present, it means the keloid is active and enlarging. This border activity may be amenable to the V beam or pulsed-dye laser.

Patients with ulceration of their keloid(s) should be checked periodically for squamous cell carcinoma (Fig. 7.9), *especially* if the ulcer does not heal with standard therapy or continues to enlarge. A biopsy may be necessary, especially if the patients' keloids were previously treated with x-ray. There is usually an ulcer surrounded by an area of dyspigmentation. Also, if the keloids take on a red-brown hue, sarcoidosis must be ruled out (Fig. 7.10).

## Therapy

The most common and easiest procedure to perform for keloid removal, regardless of race and ethnicity, is surgical excision followed by intralesional corticosteroid injections. The injections should not start until 2 weeks after suture removal or the postoperative site may dehisce. Injections should be given every 3 weeks and pressure or

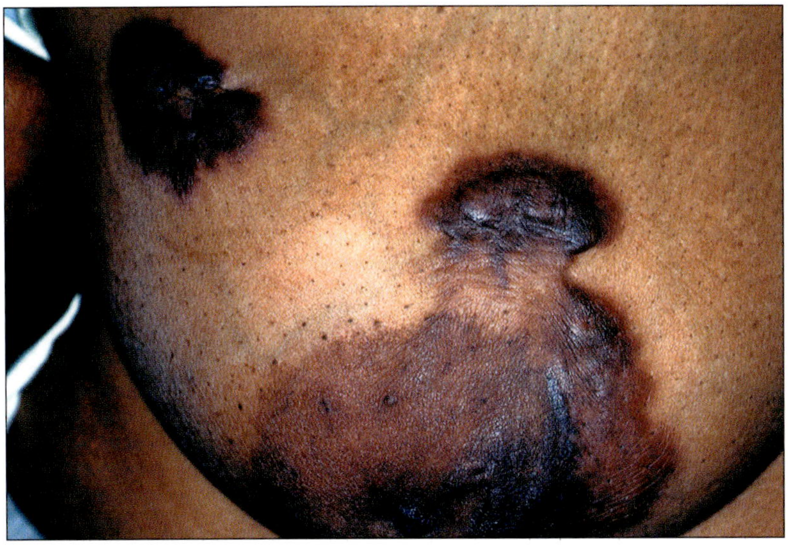

**Fig. 7.8** Keloid with erythematous border, indicating activity

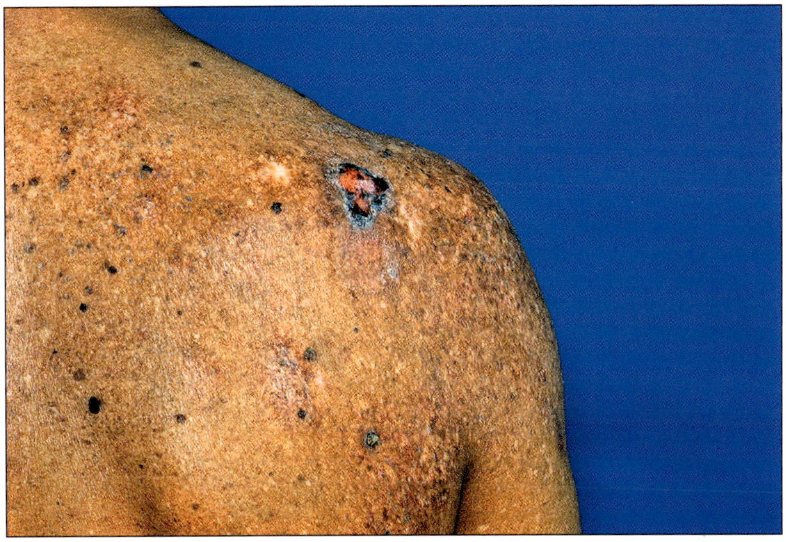

**Fig. 7.9** Squamous cell carcinoma developing in a keloid that was previously treated with x-ray

silicon applied at least 12 hours a day. The standard therapy for keloids has been discussed previously.

Patients getting their ears pierced should be concerned about keloids, especially if there is a family history of such (Box 7.1).

## Ethnic Variations

Intralesional corticosteroids are still the mainstay in treating keloids; however, patients with dark skin should be forewarned that they may develop hypopigmentation in the treated areas which may last

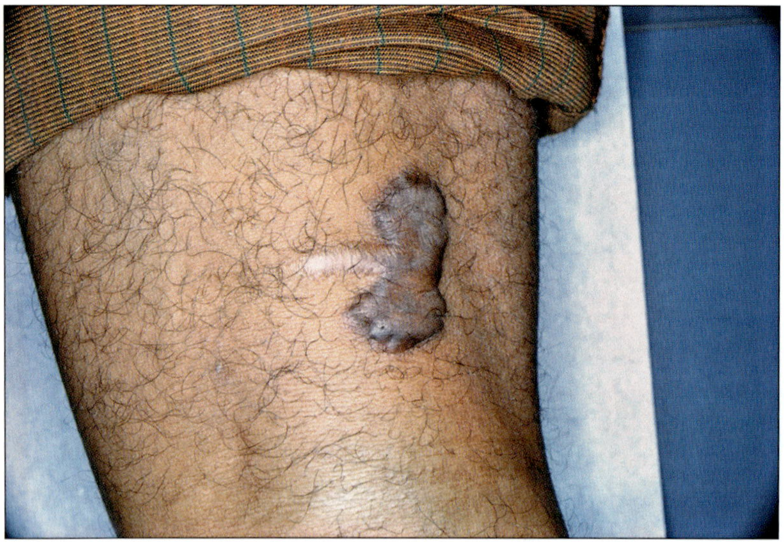

**Fig. 7.10** Sarcoid developing in a keloid

4–6 months or longer (3 mg/cc of triamcinolone acetonide or a stronger dose may cause this dyspigmentation).

Cryosurgery may be used to freeze the skin for 10–15 seconds, to cause edema of the keloid for easier injection of triamcinolone, but when cryosurgery is used to treat keloids as a monotherapy, a 30–45-second freeze is required. However, any freeze for longer than 20–25 seconds may cause hypopigmentation, which will last 1 year or longer (Fig. 7.6). Freezing for less than 20 seconds may produce cryohyperpigmentation, which will last 6–12 months. Thus, patients with dark skin should be warned prior to initiating therapy about the adverse pigment changes.

The long time use of a class I topical corticosteroid will sometimes cause hypopigmentation of the treated areas that is of greater concern in those with darker skin.

## Precipitating diseases

African-American children who have chickenpox often develop keloids in the lesion sites. Their parents should be forewarned and therapy should be started early to prevent major scarring. Herpes zoster and fraternity branding (Fig. 7.11) may also precipitate keloid formation.

Pseudofolliculitis barbae (PFB) is a common dermatologic disorder of the hair follicles that occurs most often in African-American men who shave. It may also develop in other races, women, and on any hair-bearing area that is closely and frequently shaved. The chronic inflammation stimulates collagen production, which, in turn, causes keloids (Fig. 7.12). The therapy for PFB-induced keloids is essentially the same as that for other keloids; these patients are advised to grow a beard, because this will alleviate the inflammation and camouflage excision scars. Battle and Hobbs reported that a 1064 nm Nd:YAG or

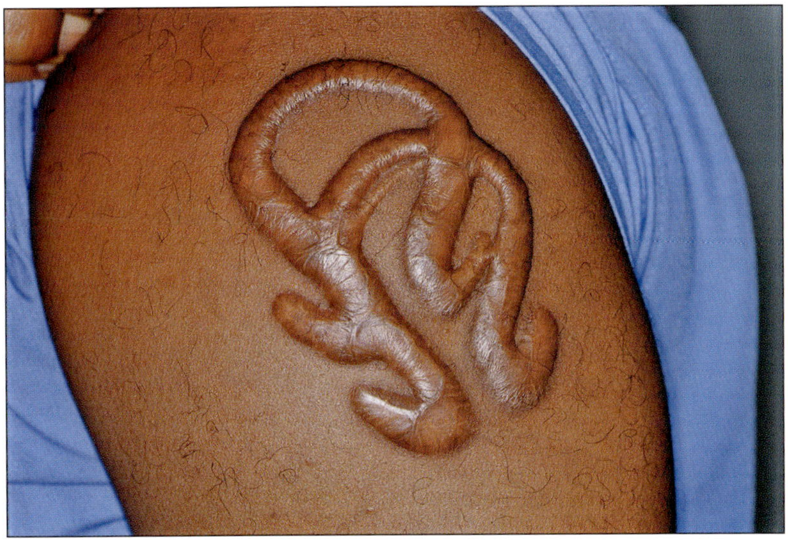

**Fig. 7.11** Keloid secondary to fraternity branding

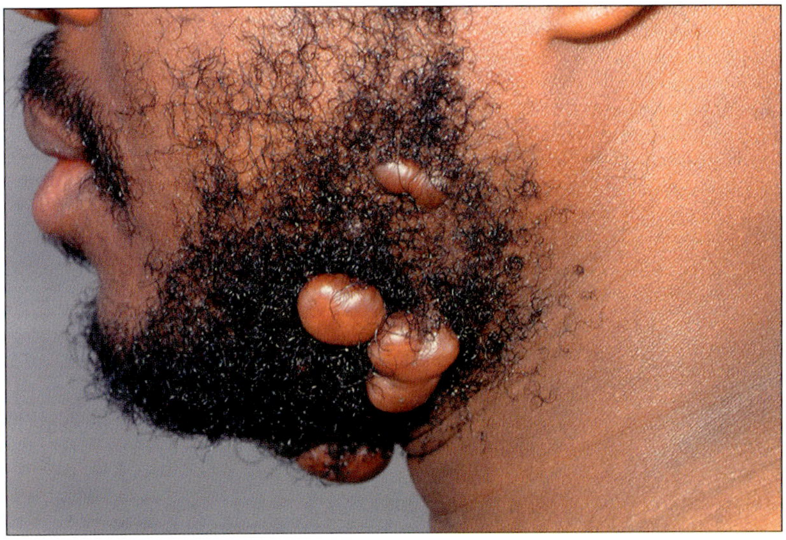

**Fig. 7.12** Keloids secondary to pseudofolliculitis barbae

pulsed-diode laser can be strongly beneficial. It will allow the older lesions to resolve and prevent new lesions from forming. This treatment can also be helpful in the treatment of acne keloidalis.

Acne keloidalis nuchae (AKN) refers to the occurrence of keloidal-like papules and plaques on the occipital scalp and posterior neck, almost exclusively in African-American men (Fig. 7.13). A study by Knable et al on the prevalence of AKN in football players at the high school, college, and professional level found that the helmets often cause a folliculitis of the nuchal area and keloidal papules developed in many African-American players but not in Caucasian players. For these patients, the problem cleared when football season was over.

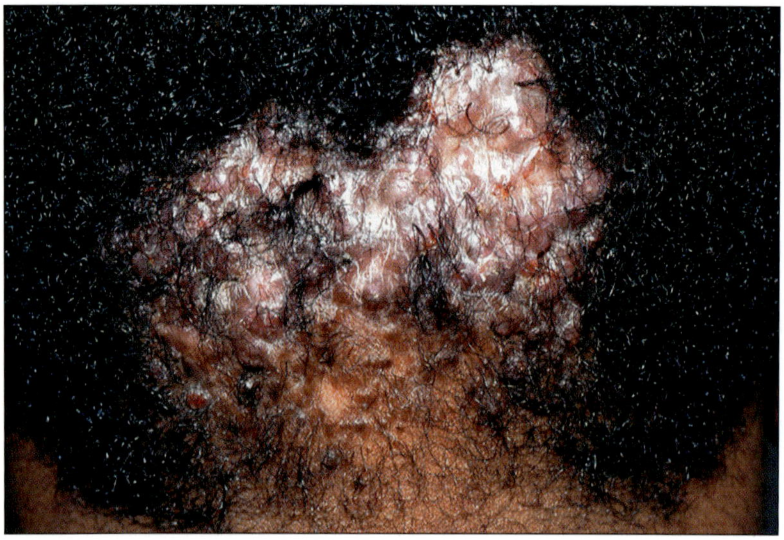

**Fig. 7.13** Acne keloidalis

## Cultural sensitivity

Cultural sensitivity helps the physician provide better service to the patients, no matter what the patient's disease.

For African-Americans it is imperative that physicians establish trust of the patient who, because of a past history of segregation, does not trust physicians. Addressing a new patient by their first name, especially if the patient is older, is considered inappropriate.

Latino patients who do not communicate well in English prefer physicians who speak Spanish. Taking a lengthy medical history with numerous questions often makes the patient feel as if the physician does not know what he or she is doing. Physicians must realize that a large percent of Latinos, especially the elderly, use herbal remedies.

Asian culture emphasizes politeness and avoidance of eye contact, which may prevent the physician from obtaining an adequate history and physical. Some patients fail to inform their physician that they are being treated by a practitioner of traditional Chinese medicine. Acupuncture, cupping, coining, and herbal medicine may be used to treat keloids and any other diseases.

## Further Reading


Battle ER Jr, Hobbs LM 2004 Laser-assisted hair removal for darker skin types. Dermatologic Therapy 17:177–183

Blackburn WR, Cosman R 1966 Histologic basis of keloid and hypertrophic scar differentiation: clinicopathologic correlation. Archives of Pathology 82:65–71

Kelly AP 2003 Keloids: pathogenesis and treatment. Cosmetic Dermatology 16-S3:29–32

Kelly AP 2003 Pseudofolliculitis barbae and acne keloidalis nuchae. Dermatology Clinics 21:645–653

Kelly AP 2004 Medical and surgical therapies for keloids. Dermatologic Therapy 17:212–218

Knable AL, Hanke CW, Gonin, R 1997 Prevalence of acne keloidalis nuchae in football players. Journal of the American Academy of Dermatology 37:570–574

# 8 Camouflage Therapy for Scars

*Neil Shear*

## Introduction

### *The problem being treated: The 'CosMedic' Clinic*

Scars are psychologically devastating for many reasons. As with any visible skin imperfection patients can be anxious, depressed, withdrawn, obsessed, or angry, but a scar is also a stigma of some trauma, many times a very unhappy one. Despite many advances in the treatment of scars, the current author has found the use of top-quality camouflage make-up to be important for patients. The make-up restores confidence, helps when other methods have failed, and provides virtually immediate benefits while waiting for other treatment options to be completed.

The current author started a camouflage make-up clinic in his university hospital ambulatory dermatology practice in 1985. It was called The CosMedic Clinic, to emphasize the cosmetic and medical aspects. The goal was to provide the powerful utility of camouflage products in a medical environment. This allowed us to use many products, thereby offering patients choices to get the best coverage. It also was more comfortable for patients with skin problems who would be embarrassed to have been treated in public. It worked better for men and children, since most camouflage options at the time were provided in 'esthetic' centers. It is also easier for patients who have scars in areas such as the legs or due to psychologically upsetting causes.

Since then the CosMedic Clinic has treated thousands of patients and many different skin problems. The most common problems are pigmentary (vitiligo, melasma). Scars are the second most common reason for referral to the clinic, and one of the most challenging to treat. Causes include surgical scars from removal of facial cancers and lymph node dissection in the neck, acne scarring, burns, and automobile accidents.

The ideal camouflage product must have many characteristics (Box 8.1). It should allow enough proper color choices so that normal skin tone can be matched with one skew, in other words, if a patient has to mix multiple colors to get the right appearance, they will not have a satisfying result. It must also be light and easy to apply; this is one of the most important goals of a make-up – that it is easy to use.

**Features of an Ideal Camouflage Product***

- A thin application is sufficient
- Water resistant or waterproof
- Provides protection (SPF >15)
- Does not need to be 'worked' before use
- Comes off easily when no longer needed
- Is available in different formulations for different body parts or needs
- Nonacnegenic
- Avoids common sensitizers
- Reasonably priced

**Only one color of the product is required for each client.*

**Box 8.1** Features of an ideal camouflage product*

The look should be natural, not heavy. It should look like there is no make-up at all.

For the first 15 years of the Clinic, a wide selection of the best-available products was used. Patients were very happy with the results, but there were major areas that needed improvement. The main issue was the mismatch of color of product with normal skin tones. Clinic physicians were able to use their clinical experience and the skills of a professional make-up chemist to develop their own product (CoverFx). The result is make-up that comes in 49 different skin tones (across all races), has superb coverage, a light and natural appearance, a sun protection factor (SPF) of at least 15, is nonacnegenic, and is easy to apply.

## Patient Selection

In many ways, make-up can be for everyone. A good product will make 'normal' skin, especially on the face, look better. A good product should also work for all skin colors and ages, and be able to reduce visible imperfections. It should be useful in all anatomical occasions. Clinic physicians have treated infants to the very elderly with camouflage make-up, and this has been appreciated by the patients. It appears that it is never too early in life, or too late, to desire a 'normal' appearance.

In Figures 8.1 and 8.2, a scar from a chest burn is covered to allow the patient to wear lower cut dresses. Burns are very difficult to cover, since they are uneven in surface, but coverage of the redness is very helpful.

In Figure 8.3 and 8.4, the CosMedic Clinic treated a young woman who had a very troubled adolescence and had self-mutilated her arms. Coverage allowed her to have the confidence to wear short-sleeved shirts and to experience the freedom to choose this option.

Eyelids can be a difficult place to apply cover effectively if the make-up is heavy. The physicians in the CosMedic Clinic have been very pleased that the very thin application required with CoverFx has allowed this area to be treated easily and with success (Figs 8.5 and 8.6).

The hand is a difficult area to treat as the appearance of veins is necessary to achieve a natural look, and the CosMedic physicians were pleased with the results in the patient in Figures 8.7 and 8.8. It should be noted that any make-up product may not hold well in circumstance where the hands are in water or when gloves are used.

The face (forehead, cheeks and jaw) are usually easy to treat with any product (Figs 8.9 and 8.10).

The legs are often undertreated and when treated, a liquid product is best. This makes application easier and the normal skin variation of the legs shows through, giving a more natural result (Figs 8.11 and 8.12).

There are patients who say they do not want or will not wear make-up. In the current author's experience, this might deter an assessment from taking place. However patients with a concern about the use of make-up (if it's not like them to wear make-up, or if they have had a

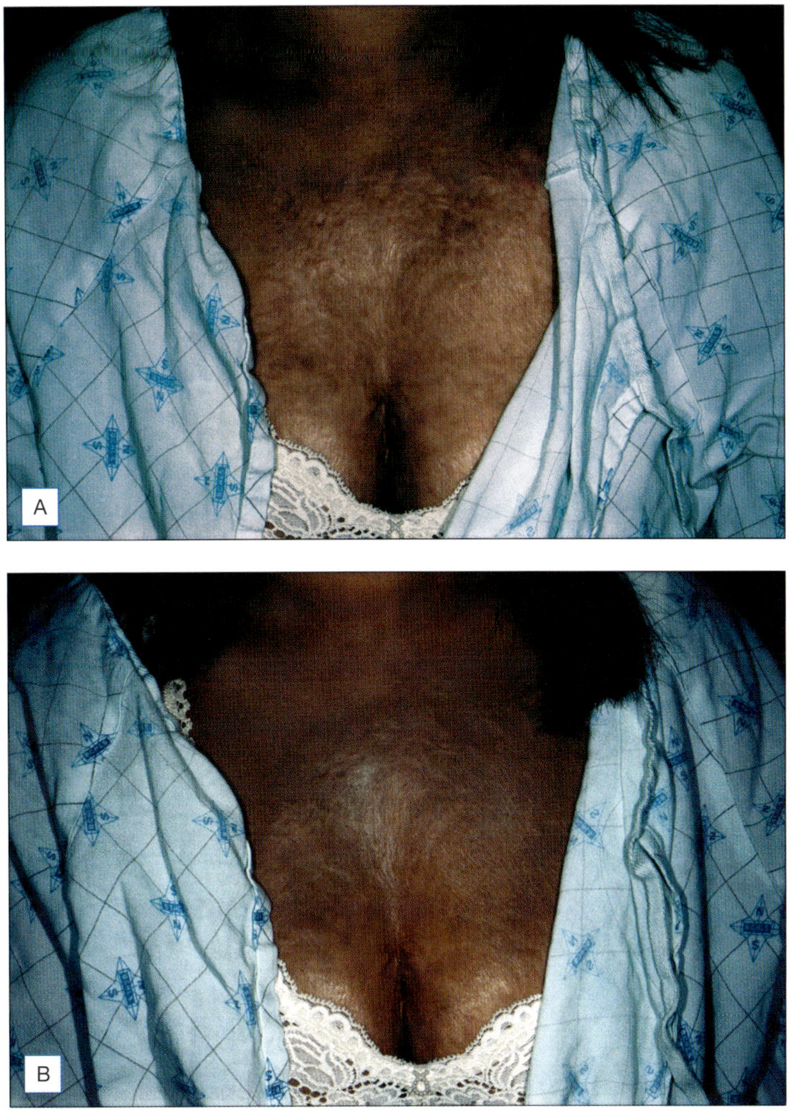

**Fig. 8.1** (**A**) Burn scar on the chest (before). This is a very challenging scar to cover (**B**) Burn scar on the chest (after). Coverage with one color of camouflage was very much appreciated by the client. The surface changes are visible, but less so than before, and the color changes are very acceptable

bad experience with make-up in the past) are usually the happiest clients after using it.

As with any topical treatment, known allergies to components of the product are a contraindication to its use.

## Expected Benefits

After the first year of operation for the CosMedic Clinic, a telephone follow up was conducted of patients who had been given color-matched

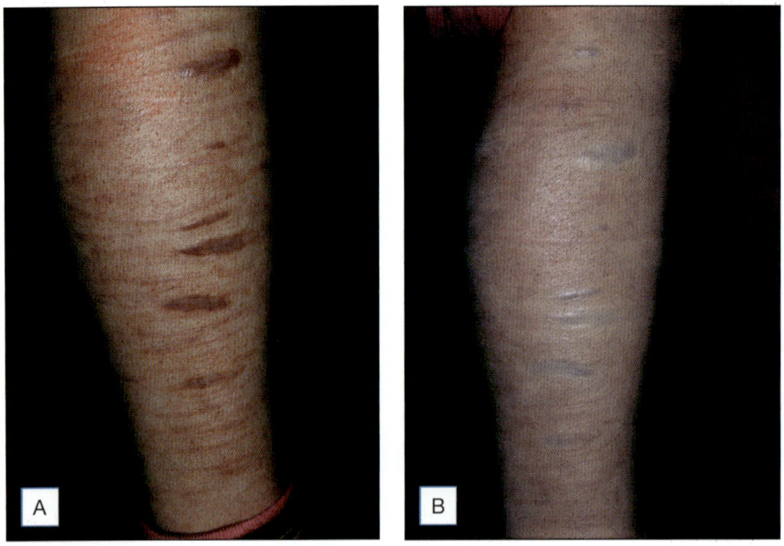


**Fig. 8.2** (**A**) Scars on the arm from self-mutilation (before). These were a severe, chronic, psychological burden. (**B**) Scars on the arm from self-mutilation (after). One color was used to give outstanding coverage. This is an example of a scar that will allow a client the freedom to wear comfortable clothing, such as a short-sleeved shirt

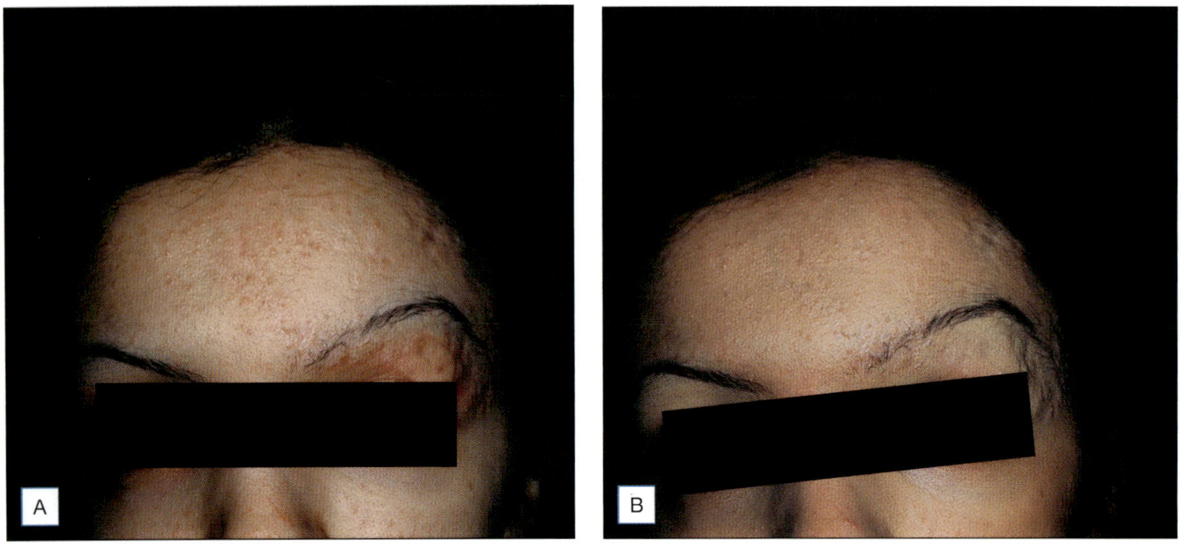


**Fig. 8.3** (**A**) Traumatic scar on eyelid (before). The redness of the scar and the acne on the forehead are both problems for this client. (**B**) Traumatic scar on eyelid (after). A single product helped with both problem areas by easily masking the redness

make-up. Over 85% were still using the make-up and were very satisfied with the results. Interestingly, some had stopped using the make-up due to concerns that it was 'medical.' Scars with dyspigmentation have shown excellent results, but scars that are very raised, or depressed, can give poorer results. Nevertheless, when an abnormal color is covered, the results are mostly quite acceptable.

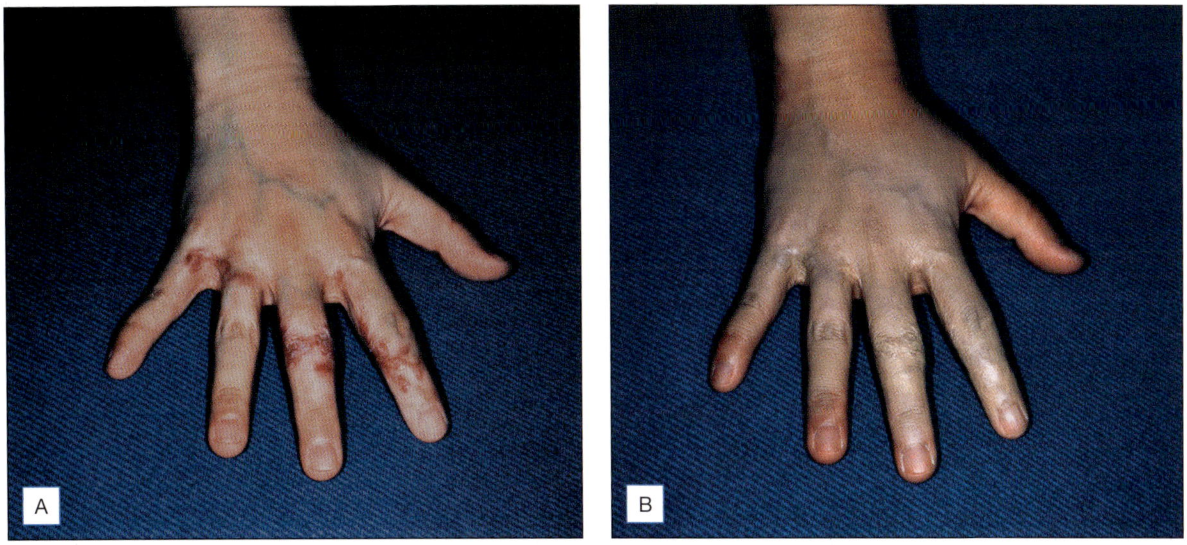


**Fig. 8.4** (**A**) Traumatic scars on the hand (before). (**B**) Traumatic scars on the hand (after). Hands are often difficult to cover, and also the temporary nature of the products is challenged by the constant wear-and-tear environment

## Comfortable, Convenient, and Safe Treatment

There are fewer treatments that are easier to use or safer than camouflage. The process is painless; there are rare cases of either contact dermatitis or acne, and if the product and service are available, it is extremely convenient. The clientele at the CosMedic Clinic are very appreciative of the 'one-stop' approach. They are assessed by a dermatologist or surgeon, and then receive the make-up match and product at the same site. The Clinic employs a cosmetician, or a nurse, who have undergone the necessary training. The product is available in the current author's hospital pharmacy.

The cost of most products is quite reasonable. For small scars, a single pot could last for 3–6 months. Powder and brushes will add to the cost, but replacements are not often needed.

## Overview of Treatment Strategy

### Treatment approach

Generally, patients access the products in either a specialized clinic (like the CosMedic Clinic, or a dermatologist's office), or they find a product at a retail outlet (such as a cosmetic counter, pharmacy, or spa). The best outcome is seen when the best product for each type of scar is used, and the service provided is of high quality. Once the correct match is made, with the right product, there should be no need for a further service component.

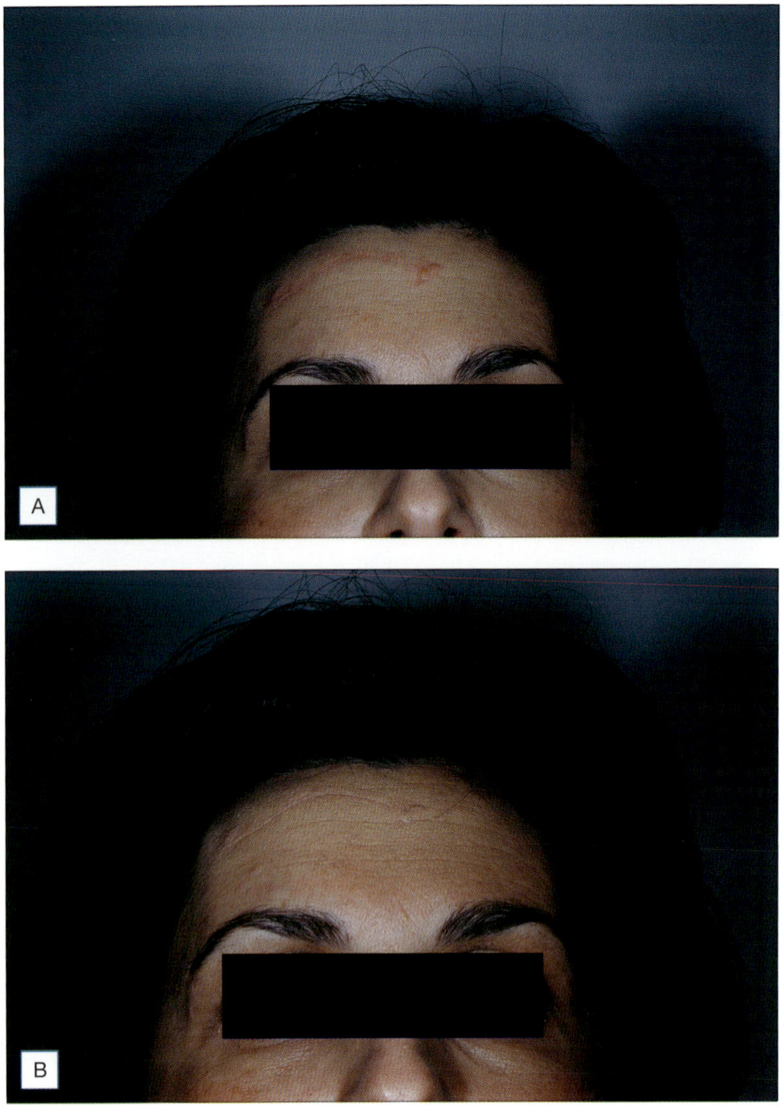

**Fig. 8.5** (**A**) Traumatic scar on the forehead (before). (**B**) Traumatic scar on the forehead (after). The simple act of covering the red makes this scar invisible at the usual distances during personal interactions. The client is now free to shop, socialize and work, without comments and questions

## Major determinants

### *Product*

A comparison of products is given in Table 8.1 based on features such as color availability, SPF, etc. It is important to note that the color availability does not necessarily mean there will be a good color match. The practitioners at the CosMedic Clinic found that color matching was one of the most important aspects of success, and that this was lacking, even in the best products. They have been amazed with the spectrum of CoverFx products. The matches are almost always right on.

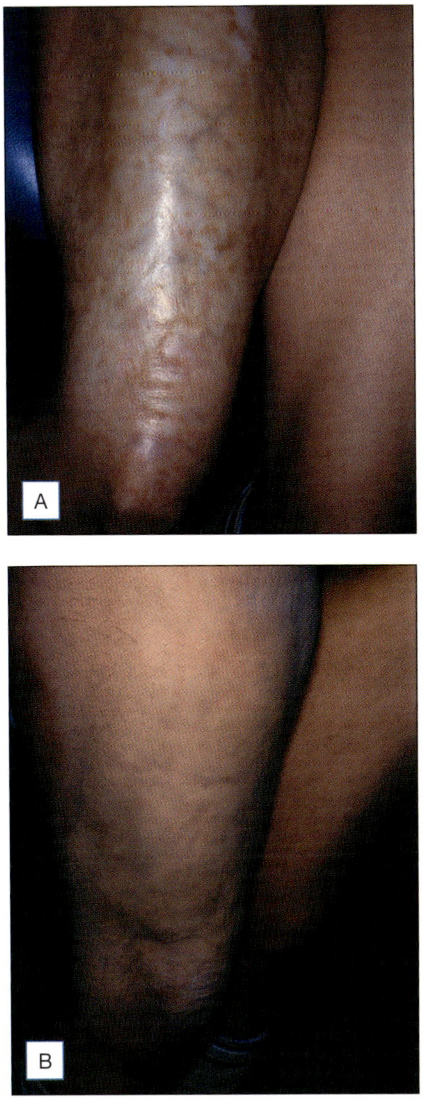


**Fig. 8.6** (**A**) Burn scar on the thigh (before). (**B**) Burn scar on the thigh (after). Scars on the legs are often not treated as aggressively as those on the face. The legs are very important and cosmetics can be very useful. The liquid formulations may work better since they are easier to apply and let some of the natural variations in the appearance show through

A good product should require very little 'work.' For example, one color should suffice, since mixing on the face will be easy for a cosmetician, but difficult for a patient. Also, the product should be soft and maintained at room temperature. It should not be necessary to warm the product before using it.

Features that help identify an 'ideal' product are listed in Box 8.2.

## *Service*

### Who should introduce the camouflage make-up?

Anyone who is comfortable with patients/clients can provide excellent color matching. The CosMedic Clinic employs mainly trained nurses and cosmeticians.

**Camouflage Technology**

- Concentrated pigment levels (20–40%)
- Film forming to build total concealment and provide all-day coverage
- Anhydrous base or external emulsion phase to provide water resistance properties
- Noncomedogenic ingredients, hypoallergenic, fragrance free and oil free to minimize adverse skin reactions
- Contains minimum of SPF 15 for environmental protection
- Emollient to aid with blending and achieve a radiant natural-looking skin finish
- Available in many shades to best match real skin tones
- Dermatologically tested

**Box 8.2** Camouflage technology

| Comparison of Most Available Products | | | | | | | | |
|---|---|---|---|---|---|---|---|---|
| **Brand/ product** | **Coverage** | **Shade range** | **Ease of application** | **Contains oil** | **Contains fragrance** | **Texture** | **SPP** | **Website address** |
| COVER FX/Total Coverage | 5 | 5 | 4 | No | No | Cream | 30 | www.coverfx.com* |
| COVER FX/Natural FX | 3 | 4 | 5 | No | No | Liquid | 15 | www.coverfx.com* |
| SHEER COVER | 3 | 2 | 4 | No | No | Powder | No | www.sheercover.com |
| JANE IREDALE/ Pure Pressed | 3 | 2 | 4 | No | No | Powder | 17 | www.lovelyskin.com |
| MAC/Studio Full Coverage | 5 | 4 | 4 | Yes | No | Cream | No | www.maccosmetics.com |
| MAKE UP FOREVER/ Camouflage Cream | 4 | 2 | 4 | Yes | No | Cream | No | www.makeupforever.com |
| DERMABLEND | 5 | 3 | 2 | Yes | Yes | Cream | No | www.dermablend.com |
| COVERMARK | 5 | 3 | 4 | Yes | Yes | Cream | 15 | www.covermark.com |
| COLORTRATION | 3 | 3 | 4 | Yes | No | Liquid | No | www.colortration.com |
| LINDA SEIDEL/ Natural Cover | 4 | 3 | 3 | Yes | No | Cream | No | www.lindaseidel.com |
| AVENE/Tinted Extreme | 1 | 1 | 4 | Yes | Yes | Cream | 50 | www.lovemarks.com |
| NEOSTRATA/Coverblend | 4 | 2 | 3 | Yes | No | Cream | 20 | www.neostrata.com/coverblend/cbd_prd_buy.asp?n=8776<br>www.neostrata.com/coverblend/cbd_prd_buy.asp?n=8776<br>www.neostrata.com/coverblend/cbd_prd_buy.asp?n=8751<br>www.neostrata.com/coverblend/cbd_prd_buy.asp?n=8772 |
| DERMACOLOUR | 5 | 5 | 4 | Yes | Yes | Cream | No | www.charlesfox.co.uk/Dermacolor/dermacolor.html |

*1, poor; 2, limited; 3, moderate; 4, good; 5, exceptional.*
**Cover Fx is available across Canada and will be in selected Nordstrum stores across the United States.*

**Table 8.1** Comparison of most available products

### Where should the make-up be distributed?

The clinic, pharmacy or spa is an ideal site, but the effective use of lighting is critical. Natural light is best, and makes it much easier to ensure that a good color match is made. A comfortable, raised stool helps bring the patient up to the cosmetician's eye level.

### What equipment is needed?

Professional boxes to hold samples are very helpful. It makes the process portable and can hold sample pots of the entire make-up product line. A brush is the best tool for application. Sponges, even excellent firm, nonlatex ones, are not as good. Sponges pull on the skin, and leave an uneven surface that does not look as natural as the results from a brush. A mirror, especially a hand-held one, is useful so that clients can see the results, but more importantly, so that they can follow the process. They will need to learn how to apply the product at home. Since the scar might be in an area that is not easily seen, say the angle of the jaw, the self-application of make-up will require some practice.

### Office set-up

If there is office space (about 100 $ft^2$ is comfortable) with outdoor natural lighting, the space can be used, even half a day per week. It takes about 20–30 minutes for each client to get the right match and feel comfortable with the proper use of the products. If the products are already sold in the office, it is easy to add a line of camouflage make-up. Even a line like CoverFx, with close to 50 colors, will require mostly 10 colors to treat most patients. This line has white, black, Asian and Mediterranean skin tone lines. The type of products needed might vary by the skin ranges seen in the practice.

If the office is not going to be used, then it may be helpful to have a sheet that directs clients to a cosmetician or retail outlet that can provide the skills and product selection required.

## *Patient interviews*

Patients may have concerns about the appropriateness of make-up, since it is not permanent, or they have tried other products and have not been satisfied. Patients with known intolerances to topical products, preservatives or vehicles, will need special attention. A nonacnegenic product will be needed for acne-prone skin.

Consultations at the Clinic include talking to the patient about their scar, the cause, any discomfort, results of previous surgical or camouflage treatments, and their feelings about make-up as an adjunct to other treatments.

Most concerns are easily answered. The product should be so light as to be unnoticeable to the client and observers. If it is not comfortable, it will not be used and while it is temporary, it is going to be easy to take off, easy to adjust colors in the future if needed, and it will always be available to help meet corrective needs in the future.

## Treatment Techniques

### Patients

Make-up works for all patients, regardless of gender, age, or race. Men and children are often the most appreciative since this type of product may never be offered to them in a normal course of events.

### Equipment

- Make-up kit box with tester samples of all colors.
- Brushes for application of make-up and brushes for fixer powder application.
- Hand-held mirror.

### Treatment algorithm

- Pick a starting color. The neck is a good site to use to see what the normal skin tone should be.
- Apply the product with a brush, with a dabbing motion. Then 'feather' the edges so that the border is not visible.
- Adjust the color if needed (darker or lighter, more or less red/yellow etc.).
- Apply the fixing powder.
- If the entire face is being treated, then consider a colored powder or bronzer, to enhance appearance.

### Troubleshooting

Trouble is a very rare occurrence. Sometimes, due to the raised nature of the scar, or uneven surface, camouflage is not appropriate. It might work better after further surgical treatments, for example, to treat hyperpigmentation. Carrying out the color match should be done early in the treatment of the patient.

### Side effects

Contact allergy to components, or an acneiform reaction, is uncommon, but is still possible.

## Further Reading

Holme SA, Beattie PE, Fleming CJ 2002 Cosmetic camouflage advice improves quality of life. British Journal of Dermatology 147:946–949

# Index

**Notes:** page numbers in **bold** refer to tables, page numbers in *italics* refer to figures


## A

abdomen, keloids, *116*
acne keloidalis nuchae (AKN), 121, *122*
acne scars, 48, *48,* 58–61, 68, *68,* 71
  keloid-type, *23, 72*
  laser therapy
    Er:YAG, 74
    extent/severity and, 80–81
  *see also* atrophic scars; inflammation/inflammatory conditions
African-American people
  acne keloidalis nuchae (AKN), 121, *122*
  children, 120
  cultural sensitivity, 122
  treatment considerations, 115–122
African-Americans
  keloid scars, 10
age
  influence on scarring, 11–13
  keloid scars, 116
  of scar, in laser treatment, 80
allogenic soft tissue fillers, **34, 35**
alphahydroxy acids (AHA), 36
amniotic fluid, 12
anesthetics, 49
  laser/energy source treatment, 82
apoptosis, 5–7
  function, **5**
  keloid fibroblasts, 4, 5
  signals, 7
Aquaphor Healing Ointment, postoperative care, 50–51
Artecoll, **34**
Artefill, **34**
Asians
  cultural sensitivity, 122
  keloid scars, 10
ataxia telangiectasia, 97
atrophic scars, 11, 58–61, 68, *68*
  laser/energy source therapy, 78
    Er:YAG laser, 74
    Nd:YAG 1320 laser, 75
  pathogenesis, 71–72
  *see also* acne scars
Autologen, **34, 35**
autologous fat injection, **34, 35**
autologous fibroblasts, **32, 34, 35**
autologous tissue fillers, **32, 34, 35**
axilla scars, *117*

## B

beta-hydroxyl acids (BHAs), 36
  advantages, 36–37
bleomycin, intralesional, 39
Bloom syndrome, 97
bolus, 90
  depth dose alterations, *92, 93*
botulinum toxin, 42
bovine collagen, **32**
bovine tissue filler, **34, 35**
brachytherapy, 90

## C

Caesarian section, keloids after, *29*
camouflage therapy, 20, 123–134
  advantages, 127
  benefits, 125–126
  cost issues, 127
  features of idea product, **123**
  patient interviews, 131
  patient selection, 124–125
  problem being treated, 123–124
  product, 129, **130,** 132
  service, 129–131
    distribution, 131
    office set-up, 131
  strategy, 127–128, 129–131
  techniques, 132
  technology, **129**
  *see also individual areas*
cancer risk
  keloids, 118, *119, 120*
  laser-induced repigmentation, 107
  radiation treatment, 102
Captique, fillers, 62
carbon dioxide laser, 73
  epidermal blister roofs, 111
  recovery time, 81
  skin type, 80
caspase family, apoptosis, 6
chemical peels, 33, 36–39
  adverse reactions, **40**
  follow-ups, **37**
  healing time, 38
  medium-depth peels, 36–37
  treatment algorithm, **38**
  types, **36**
chest burn scar, camouflage therapy, 124, *125*

chest keloids, *19, 116*
chicken pox, African-American children, 120
children
  African-American, 120
  radiation treatment, 97
clinical features, 8–11
collagen fillers, 61–62
  autologous, **32, 34, 35**
  bovine, **32, 35**
collagen vascular disease, radiation treatment, 96
compression therapy, 24–25
Cordran tape, 22
  side effects, 24
coronary bypass surgery, keloid scars after, *26*
corticosteroid injections, 25–28, 119–120
  alternative approaches, 28
  equipment, **27**
  patients, 25, 27
  pulsed-dye-laser treatment and, 87
  side effects/complications, 28
  treatment algorithm, 27–28
  treatment issues, 19
  troubleshooting, 28
'CosMedic' clinic, 123–124
cosmetic issues, 18
  surgical approaches, 45
CoverFx, 124
  products, 129
cryosurgery, *20*
  keloids, 120
cryotherapy, 30–31
  equipment, 30
  patients, 30
  treatment algorithm, 30
  trouble shooting, 30–31
cultural sensitivity, 122
Cymetra, **34, 35**

## D

deep defects
  dermal fillers, 62, *62*
  surgical approaches, 51–52
definitions, 1
dermabrader, 65
dermabrasion, 63–65
  contraindication, 65
  indications, 63
  treatment algorithm, 63–65
dermal fillers *see* fillers
dermal grafting, 63, *64*
Dermalogen, **34, 35**
dermasanding, 65
diabetic patients, treatment issues, 19
diode 1450 lasers, 74–76
DNA, radiation treatment effects, 93–94

## E

earlobe keloids, 115, *115, 116*
electrons, 90
elliptical excision techniques, 51–52
energy source treatment *see* laser/energy source treatment
epidermal blister roofs, 110–113, *111*
  complications, 111
Er:YAG laser therapy, 74
  epidermal blister roofs, 111
  recovery time, 81
  skin type, 80
erythema
  laser resurfacing, 86
  radiation treatment, 95, 101
estrogen
  influence on scarring, 13–14
  treatment issues, 19
ethnicity
  cultural sensitivity, 122
  keloid scars, 10, 119–122
  treatment considerations, 115–122
  *see also specific ethnic/cultural groups*
Excimer, 308nm, *108,* 109
Excimer 308nm laser, 106
excision therapy
  fusiform (elliptical), 51–52
  hypertrophic scars, 52
  keloids, 118–119
  punch, 59–60, *60*
  serial partial, 52
  shave, 51–52
extramarginal excision techniques, 51–52
eyelid scars, camouflage therapy, 124, *126*
eye protection, laser/energy source treatment, 82

## F

facial scars, camouflage therapy, 124
fat injection/transplantation, 63
  autologous, **32**
fibrinolysis, 2
fibroblasts, 3, 71
  autologous, **32, 34, 35**
  keloid, apoptosis, 4, 5
  radiation treatment, 99
fibrosis stimulation, dermal fillers, 62
fillers, 31–33, *62*
  collagen, **32,** 61
  indications, 61
  treatment algorithms, **34–35**
  types, **32,** 61–62
  *see also specific types*
Fitzpatrick's skin types III, 19
flip-top grafting, 111, *112*
5-fluorouracil (5-FU), intralesional, 39, 41
fractional photothermolysis, 112
fractional resurfacing, 76
fractionation, 93
  four Rs, 94
fusiform excision, 51–52, *52, 53*

## G

gene expression, apoptosis, 6–7
genetic factors
  influence on scarring, 13

genetic factors (*cont'd*)
predisposition to complications, 97
*see also* ethnicity
geometric broken-line closure (GBLC), 55, 57, *58*
Gore-Tex, **34**
grafting
dermal, 63, *64*
flip-top, 111, *112*
punch, 61, *111*
ultrathin split-thickness skin, 111
granulation, 2
gray (Gy), 93
grenz rays, 90
growth factors, 2

## H

hand scars, camouflage therapy, 124, *127*
head scars, camouflage therapy, *128*
health factors, treatment issues, 19
hematoma formation, 2
herpes simplex virus (HSV), reactivating, 85–86
history taking, laser/energy source treatment, 82
hormone replacement therapy, influence on scarring, 13–14
hormones, influence on scarring, 13–14
human skin, as dermal filler, 62
human tissue
radiation treatment effect, 93–94
sensitivity, radiation treatment, *95*
tissue strength, 3
tissue thickness, radiation treatment, 90, *91*
hyaluronic acid, 12
fillers, 61, 62
hyaluronic acid-stimulating activity (HASA), 12
hydration, 37
Hylaform, fillers, 62
hyperpigmentation
post-inflammatory, laser resurfacing, 86
transient
pulse-dye laser (PDL), 83
radiation treatment, 95
hypertrophic scars, 4, *9*
appearance, 48
clinical features, **8,** *67,* 67–68
histopathology, 8–9, *9,* **12**
keloid scars *vs.,* **117**
pathogenesis, 71
treatment
approach, *78*
corticosteroids, 25
excisional techniques, 52
laser/energy source, 77–78, 83, *84*
radiation, 89, 98–101
*see also individual methods*
hypopigmentation
causes, 105
cryotherapy, 31
laser-induced repigmentation *see* laser-induced repigmentation
radiation treatment, 101–102

## I

ice pick scars, 48, *48,* 68–69
imiquimod, 41
induration discs, *26*
infection, cryotherapy, 31
inflammation/inflammatory conditions, 2
acne scarring, *23,* 71
hyperpigmentation, 86
laser/energy source treatment, 81–82
scarless fetal wound healing, 11–12, 13
steroid treatment *see* corticosteroid injections
infrared lasers, striae distensae, 79
inherited disorders, sensitivity to x-rays, 97
interferon therapy, 41
intralesional 5-fluorouracil, 39, 41
intralesional bleomycin, 39
intralesional steroids, 119–120
Isolagen, **34, 35**
isotretinoin
laser/energy source treatment, 82
treatment issues, 19

## J

Jessner's solution, 33
advantages, 38
Juvederm, fillers, 62

## K

keloid-derived human keratinocytes (KHKs), 4
keloid fibroblasts, apoptosis, 4, 5
keloid scars, 4, *10*
acne and, *23, 72*
age and, 116
clinical features, **8,** 9–10, 68, *68*
common areas, 115–116
abdomen, *116*
chest, *19, 116*
earlobe, 115, *115, 116*
neck, *116*
differential diagnosis, 117
erythematous border, *119*
ethnicity and, 10, 119–122
histopathology, 10, *11,* **12**
hypertrophic scars *vs.,* **117**
incidence, 115
invasion, 47–48
pathogenesis, 4, 10, 71
pedunculated, *27*
postoperative, *26, 29*
recurrence
factors for, **115**
prevention, 99
sarcoid development, *120*
secondary to branding, *121*
squamous cell carcinoma, ulcerated keloids, 118, *119*
therapy, *17,* 117–119
corticosteroids, 25, 118
cryosurgery, 120
excisional techniques, 52, 118–119
intralesional corticosteroids, **27**

keloid scars (*cont'd*)
laser/energy source treatment, 77–78
radiation treatment, 89, 98–101, *100*
therapeutic gems, 118
*see also individual therapies*
*see also specific locations*
keratinocytes, 3
apoptosis, 6
keloid-derived, 4

## L

language difficulties, cultural sensitivity, 122
laser/energy source treatment, 67–88
patient selection, 69–70
practitioners, tips for, 87
recovery time, 81
repigmentation *see* laser-induced repigmentation
scarring, types, 80–81
atrophic, 78
hypertrophic, 77–78
keloids, 77–78
striae distensae, 78–79
techniques, 82–87
Er:YAG *see* Er:YAG laser therapy
expected benefits, 72–76
fractional resurfacing, 76
infrared, 79
laser resurfacing, 84–86
Nd:YAG 1320, 74–76
nonablative, 86–87
plasma rejuvenation/resurfacing, 76–77
pulsed-dye (PDL) *see* pulsed-dye laser (PDL) therapy
treatment options, **69**
treatment strategy, 77–82
approaches, 77–79
considerations, 79–82
*see also individual techniques; specific types of scar*
laser-induced repigmentation, 105–113, *106, 108*
benefits, 106–107
candidates, 105–106
contraindications, 105–106
equipment, 109
shielding, 107, *109*
side effects, 106
laser resurfacing, techniques, 84–86
Latino people, cultural sensitivity, 122
leg scars, camouflage therapy, 124
Li Fraumeni syndrome, 97
Lumenis, relume UVB hand-held phototherapy device, 109

## M

macrophages, 2
malignancy risk *see* cancer risk
mast cells, keloid scars, 10
matrix metalloproteinases, 5
melanocytes
keloid scars, 10
transplantation, 110
micronized alloderm, **32, 34, 35**
microthermal zones (MTZs), 112
monocytes, 2
radiation treatment, 99
myofibroblasts, 3

## N

Nd:YAG 1320 laser therapy, 74–76
neck keloids, *116*
neutrophils, 2
Nokor Admix needle, 58
nonablative laser, techniques, 86–87
nonmalignant systemic disorders, radiation treatment, 96
nonsilicone occlusive sheets, 22
nutritional status, treatment issues, 19

## O

occlusion therapy, 20–24
algorithm, **22**
alternative approaches, 23–24
patients, 22–23
side effects/complications, 23–24
troubleshooting, 23
oral contraception, treatment issues, 19
orthovoltage x-rays, 90

## P

*p*53 gene, apoptosis, 5
pain
corticosteroid injections, 27, 28
cryotherapy, 31
pathological features, 8–11
patient interviews, 81–82
phenol, 37
photons, 89–90
skin-sparing properties, *92*
photosensitivity, medications causing, **33**
pigmentation
hyperpigmentation *see* hyperpigmentation
hypopigmentation *see* hypopigmentation
therapy, 21
camouflage *see* camouflage therapy
laser *see* laser-induced repigmentation
plasma rejuvenation/resurfacing, 76–77
polymethylmethacrylate, **32, 34**
polytetraflouroethylene, **32, 34**
polyurethane dressing, 22
postblepharoplasty hypopigmented scar, *108*
pressure dressing, 24
postoperative care, 50
prevention, 49
programmed cell death *see* apoptosis
proliferation, 2–3
pseudofolliculitis barbae (PFB), 120–121, *121*
psychological factors, 18, 69, 123
pulsed-dye laser (PDL) therapy, 72–73, *73, 85*
corticosteroid injections and, 87
hypertrophic scars, 77–78
keloid scars, 77–78
skin type, 79–80
striae distensae, 79
techniques, 82–83

punch elevation, 60
punch excision, 59–60, *60*
punch grafting, 61, *111*
punch micrografting, 110
purpura, pulse-dye laser (PDL) therapy, 83

## R

radiation treatment, 89–103
  acute/late sequelae, 101–102
  clinical effect, 93–94
  complication risks, 96–97
  definitions, 89–90, 93–94
  dose-dependent effects, **101**
  dose distribution, *91, 92, 93*
  excision, following, 99–100, 102
  hypertrophic scars, 98–101
  keloid scars, 98–101
  normal skin effects, 94–96, *95*
  patient selection, 96–97
  targets, *100*
recovery time, laser/energy source treatment, 81
relaxed skin tension lines (RSTLs), 18–19, *46*
remodeling, 3
repigmentation, laser-induced *see* laser-induced repigmentation
Restylane, fillers, 61–62
resurfacing techniques
  fractional, 76
  laser, 84–86
  plasma, 76–77
retinoblastoma, 97
retinoic acid, topical, 41
rheumatoid arthritis, radiation treatment, 96
rolling scars, 48, *48, 58*

## S

salicylic acid, 33, 36
sarcoid development, keloid, *120*
Scarguard, 22
scar irregularization, 53–55
scarless fetal wound healing, 11–13
scarring
  abnormal scars, 3–4, **46**
    disease-related, 48
    poor healing, 47
    poorly designed, 45, 47
    traumatic, 47
    treatment approaches, **47**
  clinical, 45, 47–48
  factors affecting, 11–14
  normal scars, 3
  *see also specific types*
self-mutilation scars, camouflage therapy, 124, *126*
serial partial excision, 52
shave excision, 51
  troubleshooting, 51–52
shielding, laser-induced repigmentation, 107, *109*
silicone
  dressings, 21–22
  fillers, **32, 34, 35**
SI (Systeme International d'Unites) radiation unit, 93
skin tone, laser/energy source treatment, 70
skin type, laser/energy source treatment, 79–80, 82
soft tissue fillers *see* fillers
squamous cell carcinoma, ulcerated keloids, 118, *119*
steroid injections *see* corticosteroid injections
stretch marks (striae distensae), *29*
  laser/energy treatment, 78–79
subcision (SC), 58–59
sun exposure, avoidance, 107, 109, **109**
surgical approaches, 45–66
  acne/atrophic scar revision, 58–61
  dermabrasion, 63–65
  dermal grafting, 63, *64*
  dermasanding (manual dermabrasion), 65
  excisional techniques *see* excision therapy
  fat transplantation, 63
  general principles, 49–51
  geometric broken-line closure (GBLC), 55, 57
  patient selection, 48–49
  postoperative care, 50–51
  preoperative approach, 49
  scar irregularization, 53–55
  *see also specific techniques*
sutures, 50, *50*
syncope, cryotherapy, 31
Systeme International d'Unites (SI) radiation unit, 93

## T

tacrolimus, 41–42
tensile strength, treatment issues, 20
thigh, camouflage therapy, *129*
toxicity, radiation treatment, 94–96
transforming growth factor β (TGFβ), 4
  TGF-β1, 4, 71
    apoptosis, 5–6
    estrogen influence, 13
  TGF-β2, 4
  TGF-β3, 4
treatment, 17–43
  abnormal scars, **47**
  general approach, 49
  preventative, 20, **21**
  relative exclusion criteria, **19**
  scar types, **69**
  timing, 20
  *see also individual approaches*
triamcinolone acetonide, 25
  injecting, 118
trichloroacetic acid (TCA), 33, 36–37
tumor necrosis factor (TNF) superfamily, 6
tumors, radiation treatment, 95

## U

ultrathin split-thickness skin grafting, 111
Unna's resorcinol paste, 33
UVB lasers, repigmentation *see* laser-induced repigmentation

## V

vasculature effects, radiation, 98
verapamil, 39

## W

waterproof silicone carbide sandpaper, 65, *66*
wound healing, 1–2
full-thickness, 1–2
partial-thickness, 1
postoperative, 50
potential, 19
previously irradiated tissue, 97–98
process of, 70–71
radiation treatment, 97–98
stages, 2–3
W-plasty, 55, *57*

## Z

Zars patch, *29*
Z-plasty, 53–55, *54,* **55,** *56*
Zyderm, **34, 35**
Zyplast, **34, 35**